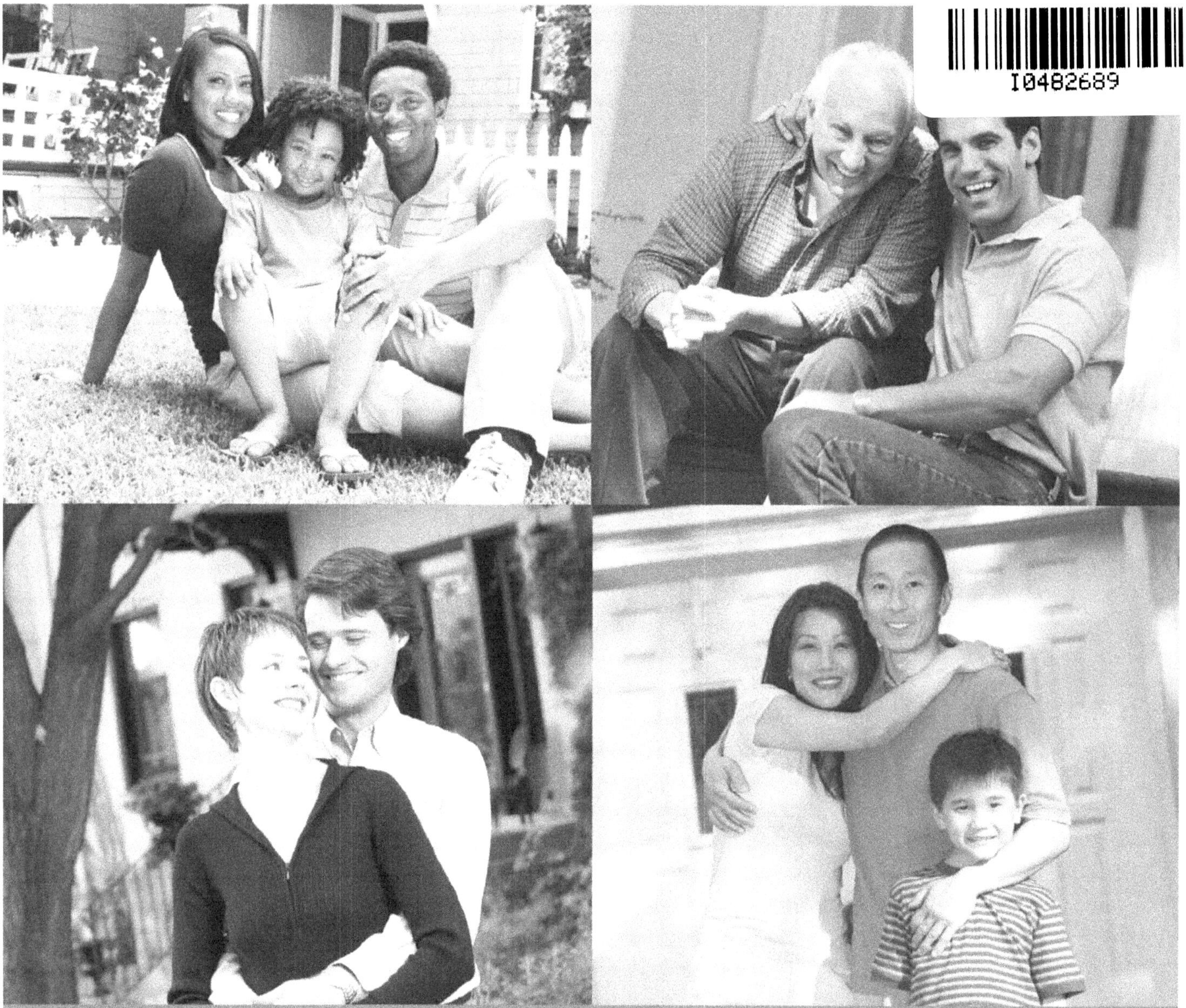

I0482689

U.S. Department of Health and Human Services
U.S. Department of Housing and Urban Development

Healthy Housing Inspection Manual

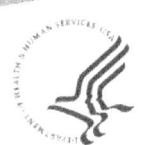

Healthy Housing
Inspection Manual

U.S. Department of Health and Human Services

U.S. Department of Housing and Urban Development

SUGGESTED CITATION: Centers for Disease Control and Prevention and U.S. Department of Housing and Urban Development. Healthy housing inspection manual. Atlanta: US Department of Health and Human Services; 2008.

For additional copies of this manual, download a PDF (http://www.cdc.gov/nceh/publications/books/ inspectionmanual) or order a CD-ROM (1-800-CDC-INFO or cdcinfo@cdc.gov). Minimally formatted word-processing files are available for programs that would like to customize the manual for their own use.

Contents

Preface

THE *HEALTHY HOUSING INSPECTION MANUAL* completes the foundation of the Centers for Disease Control and Prevention's (CDC's) Healthy Homes Initiative. The manual reflects the ongoing commitment of both CDC and the U.S. Department of Housing and Urban Development (HUD) to work together to provide local jurisdictions with tools to address housing-related health hazards. Development of this manual was supported by the HUD and CDC Healthy Homes Initiatives.

The agencies' initiatives related to healthy homes were created to develop a holistic approach to healthy housing based on the following broad objectives:

- Broaden the scope of single-issue public health and safety programs—such as childhood lead poisoning prevention, residential asthma intervention, injury prevention— to adopt a holistic approach addressing multiple housing deficiencies that affect health and safety.
- Build competency among environmental public health practitioners, public health nurses, housing specialists, housing owners, housing managers, and others who work in the community so they can incorporate healthy housing activities into their professional activities.
- Develop national healthy homes capacity through crossdisciplinary grants, contracts, and other activities at the federal, state, tribal, and community levels that research and demonstrate low-cost, effective home hazard assessment and intervention methods.
- Develop effective education and outreach materials, with a particular focus on high-risk populations, to increase public awareness of residential hazards and highlight effective actions households can take to reduce the risk for illness and injury.

The *Healthy Housing Inspection Manual* is a model reference tool that local jurisdictions or others may use as is or modify based on local needs. Use of the manual is expected to improve the effectiveness and efficiency of the public health, housing management, and workforces that identify, prevent, and control health problems associated with housing. The manual does not introduce any inspection requirements, nor does it modify any existing inspection requirements for housing agencies, residents, HUD, or CDC. The manual is not a substitute for the Federal Housing Administration (FHA) Minimum Property Standards. Finally, the manual does not propose to establish any regulatory authority for HUD or CDC with regard to residential inspection requirements.

The *Healthy Housing Inspection Manual* takes environmental health professionals and housing managers, specialists, and inspectors through the elements of a holistic home inspection. It is also a useful reference tool for nurses, outreach workers, and others who are interested in preventing illness and injury due to residential health and safety hazards.

The *Healthy Housing Inspection Manual* addresses the broad range of housing deficiencies and hazards that can affect residents' health and safety. The purpose of the manual is to

- improve communication and collaboration among public health professionals, housing professionals, property owners and property managers,
- increase the understanding of the relations among exposure to hazardous agents, conditions in the home, and adverse health outcomes, and
- improve the ability of programs to address an array of housing deficiencies in an efficient, effective, and timely manner.

HUD and CDC have also jointly developed and funded other important activities related to healthy homes, including

- a healthy housing curriculum that addresses the training needs of environmental public health practitioners, public health nurses, housing specialists, and others interested in building local capacity to address housing-related health hazards (Healthy Homes Training Center and Network, http://www.healthyhomestraining.org).

- the *Healthy Housing Reference Manual*, which gives public health and housing professionals the tools necessary to ensure that housing stock is safe, decent, and healthy for our citizens, particularly children and the elderly, who are often most vulnerable and spend more time in the home (http://www.cdc.gov/nceh/publications/books/housing/housing.htm).

FORMAT OF THIS MANUAL

HUD and CDC recommend that section 1, the Healthy Housing Model Resident Questionnaire (a voluntary health assessment), be completed first. The questionnaire should be used to collect information that cannot be determined visually. Information from the questionnaire can provide important clues that point to housing deficiencies.

SECTION 2, the Visual Assessment Data Collection Form, should be used to collect information that can be determined without asking questions of a resident. This form includes detailed assessment of exterior housing, kitchen, bathroom, and living area, as well as a general building information.

This manual also contains three supporting appendices:
- a data dictionary that defines housing deficiencies listed in the Visual Assessment Data Collection Form;
- a cross-reference to code provisions in the 2003 International Property Maintenance Code (2003 IPMC); and
- additional resources (links to environmental sampling methods and to more information about substances or issues related to healthy housing).

Section 1

HEALTHY HOMES MODEL RESIDENT QUESTIONNAIRE

Information from questionnaire responses such as these can provide important clues that point to housing deficiencies. The Healthy Homes Model Resident Questionnaire is a tool that can be adapted by local jurisdictions to meet their specific needs. Be sure to follow local jurisdiction regulations for the collection and safeguarding of personal data.

For example, jurisdictions may want to add questions about
- whether the respondent owns or rents the building/unit
- the name and contact information of the building/unit owner (rental units)
- whether the building/unit is privately owned or owned by a public housing authority
- whether the government pays some of the cost of the building/unit
- the name of the person who is responding to the questionnaire.

This questionnaire was adapted from the pediatric environmental home assessment (PEHA) created by the National Center for Healthy Housing. PEHA forms and a PEHA Nursing Care Plan can be downloaded from http://www.healthyhomestraining.org/Nurse/PEHA.htm.

The questionnaire should be used to collect information that cannot be determined without asking questions of a resident. Information that can be determined visually should be collected on the Visual Assessment Data Collection Form (Section 2).

WAS QUESTIONNAIRE ADMINISTERED?

❑Yes ❑No ❑Why not:_____ ❑Vacant

Date: _____ Name of Questionnaire Administrator: _____

Building and/or Unit Address: _____

City, State, Zip: _____

No. of persons living in unit:_____ No. of children:_____

Age of children living in unit:_____

Unit status ❑Occupied ❑Vacant

NOTE: For each questionnaire item, bolded responses indicate areas of greater concern. Responses are ordered from most potential hazard to least potential hazard.

GENERAL HOUSING CHARACTERISTICS

Type of ownership	❏Own house	❏Rental house		
Age of home	❏**Pre-1950**	❏**1950–1978**	❏**Do not know**	❏Post-1978
Floors lived in (check all that apply)	❏Basement	❏1st	❏2nd	❏3rd or higher
Heating filters changed in past 3 months	❏**No**	❏**Do not know**	❏Yes	❏Not applicable
Heating filters (type)	❏**Do not know**	❏HEPA filter	❏Not applicable	
Heating control	❏Hard to control heat	❏Easy to control heat		
Cooling method used	❏**No air conditioning**	❏Windows	❏Fans	❏Central/window air conditioner
Ventilation (check all that apply)	❏Opens window at least once a week	❏Kitchen and bathroom fans	❏Whole-house ventilation	
House/unit built with radon mitigation venting	❏**No**	❏**Do not know**	❏Yes	
Chimney inspected or cleaned in past year	❏**No**	❏**Do not know**	❏Yes	
Heating system; water heater; and other gas, oil, or coal-burning appliances serviced by a qualified technician every year	❏**No**	❏**Do not know**	❏Yes	
House/unit garbage collection	❏**Once every 2 weeks**	❏Once every week	❏Twice every week	❏Other:
House/unit water source (city water)	❏**No**	❏**Do not know**	❏Yes	
House/unit on city sewer	❏**No**	❏**Do not know**	❏Yes	
House/unit water source (individual well)[1]	❏**Yes**	❏**Do not know**	❏No	
Well tested at least once per year for coliform bacteria, nitrates, etc.	❏**No**	❏**Do not know**	❏Yes	❏Not applicable
Well test results	❏**Do not know**	❏Known (provide):		❏Not applicable
Septic tank pumped	❏**No**	❏**Do not know**	❏Date:	❏Not applicable
Well and septic system: location	❏**Do not know**	❏Known (where?):	❏Not applicable	
Well and septic system: distance between systems	❏**Do not know**	❏Known (how much?):	❏Not applicable	

[1]It would be useful to know what type of well (e.g., dug, bored, driven, drilled) and absorption system (cesspool, seepage pit, trench system, elevated mounds/sand, other) serves the house/unit. Jurisdictions may wish to think about including that information in a questionnaire or obtaining such information from other sources.

INDOOR POLLUTANTS

Mold and moisture	❑Visible water/ mold damage	❑Musty odor evident	❑Uses dehumidifier	❑No damage or odor
Any water problems?	❑Inside damp- ness during heavy rains	❑No complaints		
Pets: presence	❑Dog (#_____)	❑Cat (#_____)	❑Other: _____	❑No pets
Pets: management	❑Full access in home	❑Not allowed in bedroom	❑Kept strictly outdoors	❑Sleeping location:
Pests: cockroaches	❑Family shows evidence	❑Family reports	Present in ❑kitchen ❑bedroom ❑other	❑None
Pests: mice	❑Family shows evidence	❑Family reports	Present in ❑kitchen ❑bedroom ❑other	❑None
Pests: rats	❑Family shows evidence	❑Family reports	Present in ❑kitchen ❑bedroom ❑other	❑None
Pests: bedbugs	❑Family shows evidence	❑Family reports	Present in ❑bedroom ❑other	❑None
Pests: use of sprays, "bombs," or traps	❑Once a week	❑Once a month	❑Once a year	❑None
Lead paint hazards[2]	❑Loose, peeling, or chipping, paint, bare soil	❑Not tested/ Don't know	❑Tested, failed, and mitigated	❑Tested and passed
Asbestos: flooring that might contain asbestos[3]	❑Damaged material	❑Not tested/ Don't know	❑Tested, failed, and mitigated	❑Tested – None present
Asbestos: recently disturbed (e.g., sanding, chip- ping) flooring that might contain asbestos[3]	❑Yes	❑Don't know	❑No	
Radon	❑Failed test but not mitigated	❑Not tested/ Don't know	❑Tested, failed, and mitigated	❑Tested and passed
Tobacco smoke exposure[4]	❑Smoking allowed indoors	❑Caregiver smokes	❑Smoking only allowed outdoors	❑No smoking allowed
Other irritants	❑Potpourri, incense, candles	❑Air fresheners	❑Other strong odors (list):	❑None
Air freshener use (how often)	❑Continuously	❑Once a week	❑Once a month	❑Never
Type of cleaning	❑Sweep or dry mop	❑Vacuum (non-HEPA)	❑HEPA vacuum	❑Damp mop and damp dusting
Vacuum (how often)	❑Once a month or less	❑Once a week	❑Once a day	❑No carpet

INDOOR POLLUTANTS *(continued)*

Damp mop (how often) kitchen, bath, other hard floors	❑Never	❑Once a day	❑Once a week	❑Once a month or less
Air purifier use	❑Yes	❑No	❑Don't know	
Humidifier or dehumidifier use	**❑Reservoir not cleaned once a week**	❑Reservoir cleaned once a week		

[2]This may be an opportunity for local jurisdictions to check for Section 1018 [lead paint disclosure] compliance.
[3]9×9 older floor tile, 12×12 floor tile, sheet linoleum, mastic [glue used under floor tile or linoleum].
[4]Local jurisdictions may want to add details about where smoking is allowed (e.g., bedroom, playroom) and how many smokers live in the the house/unit.

HOME SAFETY

Poison control and other emergency response numbers	**❑Not posted by any phone**	**❑Not posted by every phone**	❑Posted by every phone	❑No land-line phone
All drugs and medicines stored in childproof cabinets out of reach of children	**❑No**	❑Yes		
Family fire escape plan	**❑None**	❑Developed and have copy available		
Safe place to meet outside in case of fire	**❑No**	❑Yes		
Home fire drill practiced in last 6 months	**❑No**	❑Yes		
Tested smoke alarms in past 6 months	**❑No**	❑Yes		
Portable space heaters always turned off when adults leave the room or go to sleep	**❑No**	❑Yes		

VOLUNTARY HEALTH ASSESSMENT DATA

Have you or anyone in the home had any of these conditions in the last 12 months or since you moved into this house/unit? Do any of these symptoms worsen when you enter the house/unit or while you are there? Do they improve after leaving? If yes, please describe.

- **ALLERGIES**
- **DOCTOR-DIAGNOSED ASTHMA**
- **ASTHMA SYMPTOMS (COUGH, WHEEZING, SHORTNESS OF BREATH, CHEST TIGHTNESS, AND PHLEGM WITHOUT A COLD OR RESPIRATORY INFECTION)**
- **CHRONIC BRONCHITIS**
- **EAR INFECTIONS (THREE OR MORE)**

- **EYE IRRITATION**
- **FREQUENT HEADACHES OR MIGRAINES**
- **HAY FEVER**
- **RESPIRATORY DISEASE**
- **SINUS PROBLEMS**
- **SKIN INFECTION/RASH**

INJURIES

During the past 3 months, did you/did you or anyone in your family have an injury where any part of the body was hurt (including burns, electric shock, or falls)?[5]

Did you talk to or see a medical professional about any of these injuries?

Please describe the circumstances or events leading to the injury, and any objects, substances, or other people involved. Include what the person was doing at the time.

POISONINGS

Have you or anyone in your family been poisoned in the house/unit by swallowing or breathing in a harmful substance such as bleach, carbon monoxide, or too many pills or prescription medications? Do not include food poisoning, sun poisoning, or poison ivy.

How many different poisonings occurred?

Please describe the circumstances or events leading to the poisoning/s, and any objects, substances, or other people involved. Include what the person was doing at the time.

Did you talk to or see a medical professional about any poisonings?

Have any children <6 years of age in the house/unit been tested for lead poisoning?
If yes, what were the test results?

Is the gas stove or oven ever used to heat the home?

Do you use an unvented space heater or fireplace? How often? What type of fuel do these items use?

---

[5]*Jurisdictions may wish to consider that some of these responses could be a result of behavior issues rather than structural issues.*

OTHER ISSUES

What is the occupation of adults in the household?

If residents are responsible for maintaining the swimming pool/hot tub, do you have the required water testing equipment? Are pool chemicals stored safely?

If you have firearms in your house/unit and young children live in or visit the house/unit, do the firearms have trigger locks or are they locked away and inaccessible to children?

Are bathroom and kitchen exhaust fans used often?

Section 2

HEALTHY HOMES VISUAL ASSESSMENT DATA COLLECTION FORM

The Healthy Homes Visual Assessment Data Collection Form is a tool that can be adapted by local jurisdictions to meet their specific needs.

The visual assessment should be used to collect information that can be determined without asking questions of a resident. Information that cannot be determined visually should be collected on the Healthy Homes Model Resident Questionnaire (Section 1).

The visual assessment form and accompanying description of health and safety conditions (Appendix 1) are adapted from the HUD Public Housing Assessment System (PHAS) and its Physical Assessment Subsystem (PASS) as well as from inspection protocols used by HUD healthy homes program grantees.

Date of Assessment _____

Building and/or Unit Street Address _____

City/State/Zip Code _____

Name of Data Collector _____

Signature _____

WEATHER CONDITIONS:

❑ Dry   ❑ Rain today or recently   ❑ Snow today or recently

Temperature: _____°F

FRONT DOOR OF UNIT FACES:

❑ North   ❑South   ❑East   ❑ West

TYPE OF UNIT BEING ASSESSED:

❑Single-family ❑Duplex   ❑Triplex   ❑Fourplex

❑Townhome   ❑Low-rise   ❑High-rise   ❑Other
                (1–3 floors) (4+ floors)

UNIT STATUS:

❑Occupied   ❑Vacant

INSTRUCTIONS FOR VISUAL ASSESSMENT OBSERVATIONS

- Select only one answer per question. If more than one answer is possible, record the most severe hazard and note the others in the comments section at the end of each section.

- Complete one set of "site" observations for each building or housing development.

- Complete one set of "exterior and building system" observations for each building.

- Complete one set of "common area" observations for each building. Do not complete the common area section if no common area exists.

- Complete one set of "unit" and "other" observations for each housing unit inspected.

- Document deviations from inspection protocol in the comments section space (e.g., units not available for inspection)

- Specific locations of specific hazards can be recorded in the comments section if desired.

For each assessment item, bolded responses indicate areas of greater concern. Imminent health and safety hazards appear in red.

Each response is defined. There is one response for each item. For descriptions of health and safety conditions and cross references to the 2003 IPMC, see Appendix 1.

This inspection protocol does not establish legal and/or complete compliance with local, state, federal or other applicable housing, building, health, safety or other applicable policies, codes, regulations, statutes and laws.

MAJOR VISUAL ASSESSMENT AREAS

SITE (ITEMS 1–29)

Items to inspect in this category are

- Fencing and Gates
- Grounds or Pavement
- Children's Play Areas
- Other

A comment area for the site category is also included in this section.

FENCING AND GATES

Site 1. Damaged/Falling/Leaning/Deteriorated Paint

❑Damaged but not functional or deteriorated paint in an area larger than 20 square feet: An exterior fence or gate is so damaged that it does not function as it should. An exterior fence, security fence, or gate is damaged and does not function as it should or could threaten safety or security.

❑No fencing or gates present

❑Damaged but functional; no deteriorated paint areas larger than 20 square feet: An exterior fence, security fence, or gate shows signs of deterioration, but still functions as it should, and it presents no risk to security or safety

❑No damage

Site 2. Holes or Openings in Soil Below Fence

❑≥6 square inches

❑<6 square inches

❑No holes or not applicable

GROUNDS OR PAVEMENT

Site 3. Areas of Erosion

❑Large erosion (depression, rut or groove more than 8 inches wide by 5 inches deep):
Runoff has extensively displaced soil, which has caused visible damage to structures
-OR-Advanced erosion threatens the safety of pedestrians or makes an area of the grounds unusable
-OR-There is a rut larger than 8 inches wide by 5 inches deep
-OR-There is extensive ponding
-OR-Water or ice has collected in a depression or on ground where ponding was not intended

❑Pooling of water (small erosion; depression, rut or groove less than 8 inches wide by 5 inches deep):
Erosion has caused surface material to collect, leading to a degraded surface that would likely cause water to pool in a confined area, especially next to structures, paved areas, or walkways, or a small rut/groove is 6–8 inches wide and 3–5 inches deep

❑No erosion

Site 4. Overgrown Vegetation

❏ **Vegetation has damaged building.** Plants have visibly damaged a component, area, or system of the property or have made them unusable/impassable. Vegetation is extensive and dense; it is difficult to see broken glass, holes, and other hazards.
-OR-Vegetation penetrates an unintended surface—buildings; gutters; fences/walls; roofs; heating, ventilation, and air conditioning units (HVAC); etc.
-OR-Vegetation is producing excessive moisture that may lead to mold or mildew on nearby exterior building surface
-OR-Tree is in danger of falling

❏ **Vegetation is present or contacts building, but no damage:** Extensive, dense vegetation obstructs the intended path of walkways or roads, but the path is still passable
-OR-Vegetation is present but causes no problem

❏ No vegetation present

Site 5. Graffiti

❏ **6 or more places:** Graffiti in 6 or more places

❏ **2–5 places:** Graffiti in 2–5 places

❏ **One place:** Graffiti in one place

❏ No graffiti

Site 6. Litter

❏ **Excessive:** More than 10 large trash or litter items

❏ **Slight or Moderate:** 2–10 large trash or litter items

❏ **None:** Fewer than 2 large trash or litter items

Site 7. Cracks in Pavement

❏ **≥¾ inch, hinging/tilting, or missing section(s) that affect traffic ability over more than 5% of the property's parking lots/driveways/roads or that cause trip hazards:** major trip hazard

❏ **<¾ inch displacement (vertical height):** minor trip hazard

❏ No cracks: level

Site 8. Fire Ants/Mounds or Harmful Insects

❏ **Yes:** Presence of fire ants/mounds or harmful insects

❏ No: Fire ants/mounds or harmful insects not seen

Site 9. Containers That Hold Water

❏ **Yes:** Presence of water-holding containers conducive to mosquito breeding

❏ No: Water-holding containers not present

CHILDREN'S PLAY AREAS

Site 10. Equipment

❏Equipment that poses an immediate threat: **REPORT TO BUILDING MANAGEMENT/OWNER IMMEDIATELY AND RECORD SPECIFICS IN THE COMMENTS SECTION**

❏≥50% of surface area broken/damaged: Most of the equipment (50% or more) does not operate as it should, but poses no safety risk

❏<50% of surface area broken/damaged: Less than half of the equipment does not operate as it should, but poses no safety risk

❏No play equipment observed (skip to Site 21)

Site 11. Paint Condition

❏Deteriorated paint on ≥50% of surface area of play area equipment

❏Deteriorated paint on <50% of surface area of play area equipment
-OR-No deteriorated paint on play area equipment

Site 12. Bare Soil

❏≥9 square feet of bare soil present in play area

❏<9 square feet of bare soil present in play area

Site 13. Injury-absorbent Surface Depth

❏No: No injury-absorbent surface under playground equipment or injury-absorbent surface depth less than 12 inches

❏Yes: Injury-absorbent surface under playground equipment at proper depth (at least 12 inches)

13b. Surface type: _____

Site 14. Deteriorated Injury-absorbent Surface

❏Yes: Injury-absorbent surface ≥50% deteriorated

❏Yes: Injury-absorbent surface <50% deteriorated

❏No deterioration

Site 15. Fencing and Gates

❏Damaged, not functional: An interior fence or gate is so damaged that it does not function as it should. An exterior fence, security fence, or gate is damaged and does not function as it should or could threaten safety or security.

❏Damaged, but functional: An exterior fence, security fence, or gate shows signs of deterioration, but still functions as it should, and it presents no risk to security or safety

❏No damage

❏No play area fencing/gates

Site 16. Condition

❑Refuse, animal feces, broken glass/sharp edges, or holes/trip hazards observed

❑No refuse, animal feces, broken glass/sharp edges, or holes/trip hazards observed

Site 17. Exposed Bolts

❑Yes: Exposed bolts are found on the playground equipment

❑No: Playground equipment does not have exposed bolts

Site 18. Hanging or Choking Hazards

❑Yes: Hanging and/or choking hazards on playground equipment

❑No: No hanging and/or choking hazards present on playground equipment

Site 19. Open "S" Hooks

❑Yes: Open "S" hooks on swings or other playground equipment

❑No: No open "S" hooks on swings or other playground equipment

Site 20. Pinch Hazards

❑Yes: Pinch hazards on playground equipment

❑No: No pinch hazards on playground equipment

OTHER

Site 21. Refuse Disposal

❑Wall or roof for outdoor enclosed area is leaning or collapsed
   -OR-Concrete slab deteriorated

❑Collection area overflowing: Area is too small to store refuse until pickup
   -OR-Garbage cans are overflowing

❑No exterior refuse disposal

❑Refuse properly contained

Site 22. Retaining Walls

❑Severe deterioration/safety risk: A retaining wall is damaged and does not function as it should or is a
   safety risk

❑Some deterioration: A retaining wall shows some signs of deterioration, but it still functions as it should,
   and it is not a safety risk

❑No deterioration

❑No retaining walls present

Site 23. Standing Water

❑Yes: Storm drainage areas (e.g., ditches) have standing water

❑No: No standing water in storm drainage areas

NOTE: This does not include stormwater detention basins, which are addressed in Site 24 and 25.

Site 24. Storm Drainage

❏**Completely blocked:** The system is completely blocked or a large segment of the system has failed because a large quantity of debris has caused: backups into adjacent area(s)
-OR-Runoffs into areas where runoffs are not intended

❏**Partially blocked:** The system is partially blocked by a large quantity of debris, causing backup into adjacent area(s)

❏**No designed storm drainage**

❏No obstructions

Site 25. Outdoor Water

❏**Yes:** Pond/lake/stream

❏**Yes:** Drainage reservoir

❏No: No other water on site

Site 26. Outdoor Water: Drainage Reservoir Fencing

❏**No:** Reservoir not fenced

❏**Yes:** Reservoir fenced but fence needs repair

❏**Yes:** Reservoir fully fenced and fence intact

❏Not applicable: No drainage reservoir

Site 27. Septic Tank

❏**Moist ground in septic tank area:**
IMMINENT HEALTH HAZARD: REPORT TO BUILDING MANAGEMENT/OWNER IMMEDIATELY AND RECORD SPECIFICS IN THE COMMENTS SECTION

❏No evidence of excessive ground moisture

❏No septic tank present

Site 28. Walkways/Steps/Hand Railing

❏**Missing or damaged or loose:** A hand rail for four or more stairs is missing, damaged, loose, or otherwise unusable; hand rail only present on one side, visible faults in the pavement: longitudinal, lateral, alligator, etc.
-OR-Pavement that sinks or rises because of the failure of sub-base materials. Five percent or more of the walkways must be impacted—50 out of 1,000 square feet, for example. Relief joints are there by design; do not consider them cracks. When observing traffic ability, consider the capacity to support pedestrians, wheelchairs, and people using walkers. Cracks greater than ¾ inch, hinging/tilting, or missing section(s) that affect traffic ability over more than 5% of the property's walkways/steps.

❏No damage

❏No walkway/steps

Site 29. Large Trees

❏Hanging over unit and touching unit

❏Well maintained: Trimmed back from unit

❏No large trees present

COMMENTS, SITE SECTION

BUILDING EXTERIOR (ITEMS 30–62)

Items to inspect in this category are

- Doors
- Fire Escapes
- Foundations
- Lighting
- Roofs
- Walls
- Windows

A comment area for the building exterior category is also included in this section.

Exterior 30. Building Access for the Disabled

❑ **Building is not accessible for the disabled**

❑ Building is accessible for the disabled

❑ Not applicable (single-family unit with no disabled residents)

DOORS

Exterior 31. Damaged Frames/Threshold/Lintels/Trim

❑ **At least one fire/emergency door not working** or cannot be locked because of damage to the frame, threshold, lintel, or trim. This also includes the main front door.

❑ **At least one door not working** or functioning or cannot be locked because of damage to the frame, threshold, lintel, or trim

❑ No damage

NOTE: This does not include damage to door hardware (locks, hinges, etc.), which is addressed in Exterior 32.

Exterior 32. Damaged Hardware/Locks

❑ **One or more door's panic hardware does not function as it should**
-OR-One entry door or fire/emergency door does not function as it should or cannot be locked because of damage to the door's hardware

❑ **One or more doors cannot be locked** and does not function as it should or cannot be locked because of damage to the door's hardware

❑ No damage

Exterior 33. Damaged Surface

❑ **≥1 inch diameter:** One door has a hole or holes larger than 1 inch in diameter, significant peeling/cracking/no paint, rust that affects the integrity of the door surface, or broken/missing glass
-OR-One entry door or fire/emergency door has a hole or holes with a diameter ranging from ¼ inch to 1 inch

❑ **¼ inch–1 inch diameter:** One door has a hole or holes with a diameter ranging from ¼ inch to 1 inch
❑ No damage

Exterior 34. Screen/Storm Doors Damaged/Missing

❏Security door inoperable

❏**Missing screen or glass:** At least one screen door or storm door is damaged or is missing screens or glass—shown by an empty frame or frames

❏**Missing door:** There must be evidence that a screen/storm/security door existed

❏No damage

Exterior 35. Deteriorated/Missing Caulking/Seals/Flashing

❏**Missing or damaged caulk, seals, or flashing:** The seals/caulking is missing on one entry door, or they are so damaged that they do not function as they should

❏No missing or damaged caulk, seals, or flashing

❏Not designed to have seals, caulk, or flashing

Exterior 36. Missing Doors (In Exterior Doorway)

❏**Yes:** One or more doors is missing

❏No: All doors are present

FIRE ESCAPES

Exterior 37. Egress

❏**Fire escape blocked** or otherwise not functioning

❏No fire escape

❏Fire escape functioning and not blocked

Exterior 38. Components

❏**Ladder, railing, stair missing (or not operational):** Any of the functional components that affect the function of the fire escape (for example, one section of a ladder or a railing) are missing

❏No fire escape

❏No missing components

Exterior 39. Fire Escape/Emergency Egress

❏**No:** No fire escape for basements with bedrooms and finished living spaces

❏Yes: At least one fire escape for basements with bedrooms and finished living spaces

❏Not applicable

FOUNDATIONS
Exterior 40. Foundation Type

❑Slab

❑Crawl space

❑Basement

❑Cellar

Exterior 41. Cracks/Gaps

❑≥⅛ inches wide × ⅛ inches deep × 6 inches long: Cracks more than ⅛ inch wide by ⅛ inch deep by 6 inches long
-OR-Large pieces—many bricks, for example—are separated or missing from the wall or floor
-OR-Large cracks or gaps (a possible sign of a serious structural problem)
-OR-Cracks run the full depth of the wall, providing opportunity for water penetration
-OR-Sections of the wall or floor are broken apart

❑<⅛ inches wide × ⅛ inches deep × 6 inches long: Cracks smaller than these dimensions

❑No cracks/gaps: No signs of deterioration

Exterior 42. Spalling/Exposed Rebar

❑≥50%: Obvious, significant spalled area(s) are affecting 50% or more of any foundation wall
-OR-Spalling is exposing any reinforcing material (rebar or other material)

❑10 to <50%: Obvious, large spalled area(s) are affecting 10%–50% of any foundation wall

❑<10%

❑Not applicable (no foundation)

LIGHTING
Exterior 43. Fixtures/Bulbs

❑≥20% broken/inoperable
-OR-The condition constitutes an obvious safety hazard: **REPORT TO BUILDING MANAGEMENT/ OWNER IMMEDIATELY AND RECORD SPECIFICS IN THE COMMENTS SECTION**

❑<20% broken/inoperable, but this does not constitute an obvious safety hazard

❑No exterior lighting

❑No broken/inoperable fixtures/bulbs

ROOFS

Exterior 44. Damaged/Clogged Drains (Roofs)

❏ **Fully clogged:** Drain is so damaged or clogged with debris so the drain no longer functions (shown by ponding)

❏ **Partially clogged:** Debris around or in a drain, but no evidence of ponding
-OR-Drain is damaged or partially clogged with debris, but the drain system still functions and there is no evidence of ponding

❏ No clog

❏ No drain

NOTE: This does not include gutters and downspouts, which are addressed in Exterior 48.

Exterior 45. Chimney Clearance

❏ **All chimneys do not have good clearance above roof line:** Chimney height is less than 3 feet above the highest point where the chimney penetrates the roofline

❏ **All chimneys have good clearance above roof line:** Chimney height is more than 3 feet above the highest point where the chimney penetrates the roofline

❏ No chimneys

Exterior 46. Damaged Soffits/Fascia/Flashing

❏ **Missing or damaged with water intrusion:** Soffits or fascia that should be there are missing or so damaged that water penetration is visibly possible

❏ **Some cracks but no water intrusion:** Damage to soffits or fascia, but no obvious opportunities for water penetration

❏ No damage

Exterior 47. Vents

❏ **Missing or major damage:** Vents are missing or so visibly damaged that further roof damage is possible.

❏ **Some damage:** The vents are visibly damaged, but do not present an obvious risk to promote further roof damage

❏ No damage

NOTE: This does not include exhaust fans on the roof or soffit vents, which are addressed in Building Systems 65.

Exterior 48. Gutters/Downspouts

❏ **Some components missing:** Splashblocks or other components are missing. Drainage system components are missing, causing visible damage to the roof, structure, exterior wall surface, or interior.

❏ **Some components damaged:** Splashblocks or other components are damaged. Drainage system components are damaged, causing visible damage to the roof, structure, exterior wall surface, or interior.

❏ **Both:** Some components are missing and some are damaged

❏ No damaged or missing

Exterior 49. Gutters/Downspout Discharge

❑Less than 2 feet from building foundation or grading causes water to pool near foundation

❑Discharges directly to storm water system

❑More than 2 feet from building and grading is sloped away from foundation

NOTE: This does not include clogged drains, which are addressed in Exterior 44.

Exterior 50. Shingles or Tiles or Other Roofing Material

❑≥100 square feet of shingle or tile damage

❑One shingle to less than 100 square feet of shingle, tile, or roofing material damage

❑One shingle or tile missing/damaged (<1 square foot)

❑No missing or damaged shingles, tiles, or roofing material

WALLS

Exterior 51. Primary Exterior Wall Surfaces

❑Brick
❑Stucco
❑Wood
❑Stone
❑Cement/concrete block
❑Asbestos
❑Vinyl

❑Other: _____

Exterior 52. Secondary Exterior Wall Surfaces

❑Brick
❑Stucco
❑Wood
❑Stone
❑Cement/concrete block
❑Asbestos
❑Vinyl

❑Other: _____
❑Not applicable

Exterior 53. Wall Cracks and Gaps

❑≥⅛ inches wide × ⅛ inches deep × 6 inches long: Crack(s) more than ⅛ inch wide by ⅛ inch deep by 6 inches long

-OR-evidence of moisture intrusion

-OR-Pieces—many bricks, for example—are separated from the wall

-OR-Crack(s) run the full depth of the wall, providing opportunity for water penetration

-OR-Sections of the wall are broken apart

❑<⅛ inches wide × ⅛ inches deep × 6 inches long: Crack(s) less than ⅛ inch wide by ⅛ inch deep by 6 inches long and no evidence of moisture intrusion

❑No cracks/gaps

Exterior 54. Damaged Chimney

❑Chimney separated from wall

❑Holes >4 inches × 4 inches: The surface of the chimney shows surface damage on more than one piece of wall—a few bricks or a section of siding, for example

-OR-The surface of the chimney has holes that affect an area larger than 4 inches by 4 inches

❑Both holes and separation

❑Holes observed, total area of opening <4 inches × 4 inches

❑No damage or no chimney required

Exterior 55. Wall Surface Deterioration

❑≥8½ × 11 inches: A missing piece—a single brick or section of siding, for example—or a hole larger than ½ inch in diameter

-OR-Deterioration affects an area larger than 8½ inches by 11 inches

-OR-Deterioration exposes any reinforcing material (rebar)

-OR-There is a hole of any size that completely penetrates the exterior wall

-OR-Wall surfaces out of plumb (≥1 inch in 20 feet)

-OR-Wall surface out of horizontal alignment (≥1 inch in 20 feet)

❑Up to 8½ inches × 11 inches: A missing piece—a single brick or section of siding, for example—or a hole smaller than ½ inch in diameter

-OR-Deterioration affects an area up to 8½ inches by 11 inches

❑No missing pieces/holes/spalling

Exterior 56. Masonry Caulking and/or Mortar

❑≥12 inches missing/damaged: Mortar is missing around more than one contiguous masonry unit

-OR-Deteriorated caulking in an area longer than 12 inches

❑<12 inches missing/damaged: Mortar is missing around a single masonry unit

-OR-Deteriorated caulk is confined to less than 12 inches

❑No damage or no caulking/mortar required

Exterior 57. Wall/Soffit/Fascia Paint/Water Damage

❑**≥20 square feet:** More than 20 square feet of building exterior walls affected

❑**<20 square feet, but some staining:** Less than 20 square feet of building exterior walls affected

❑No water stains/peeling or no paint required (e.g., brick walls)

WINDOWS

Exterior 58. Window Panes

❑**One or more missing or broken:** A glass pane is missing
  -OR-A glass pane is cracked or broken AND sharp edges are seen

❑**Both broken and missing:** More than one window has broken and missing glass panes

❑**One or more cracked:** A glass pane is cracked but no sharp edges are seen

❑None broken, cracked, or missing

Exterior 59. Screens

❑**1 or more screens damaged:** One or more screens in one building are punctured, torn, or otherwise damaged

❑**1 or more screens missing:** Do not cite this if the window is not designed to have a screen

❑**Both damaged and missing:** One or more screen damaged or missing

❑No screens damaged or missing or no screen required

Exterior 60. Sills/Frames/Lintels/Trim

❑**Major damage, missing or exposed interior wall, not weathertight:** Sills, frames, lintels, or trim are missing or damaged, exposing the inside of the surrounding walls and compromising its weather tightness

❑**Some damage, but no wall exposed, still weathertight:** Damage to sills, frames, lintels, or trim, but nothing is missing. The inside of the surrounding wall is not exposed. No impact seen on either the functioning of the window or weather tightness.

❑No damage

Exterior 61. Caulking/Seals/Glazing Compound

❑**Missing or deteriorated, leaks or damage present:** There are missing or deteriorated caulk or seals—with evidence of leaks or damage to the window or surrounding structure

❑**Missing/deteriorated, but no leaks or damage:** Most of the window shows missing or deteriorated caulk or glazing compound, but there is no evidence of damage to the window or surrounding structure or leaks

❑Not missing or deteriorated

Exterior 62. Window Assembly or Trim Paint

❏≥50%: Peeling paint or a window that needs paint on more than 50% of the painted surface

❏10% to <50%: Peeling paint or a window that needs paint on between 10%–50% of the painted surface

❏<10%, but some non-intact: Peeling paint or a window that needs paint on less than 10% of the painted surface

❏All intact: All paint on exterior windows is intact or no paint is required (e.g., aluminum or vinyl windows)

COMMENTS, EXTERIOR SECTION

BUILDING SYSTEMS (ITEMS 63–81)

NOTE: This section is for multihome sites only. If this is a single-family home, skip to Item 103.

Items to inspect in this category include
- Electrical systems
- Fire protection
- HVAC

A comment area for the building systems category is also included in this section.

Building Systems 63. Central Water Supply or Sewage System
❑ Water leaks observed: If leaking water is a safety concern (i.e., is leaking on or near electrical equipment), **REPORT IT TO BUILDING MANAGEMENT/OWNER IMMEDIATELY AND RECORD SPECIFICS IN THE COMMENTS SECTION**

❑ No water leaks observed

Building Systems 64. Outside Water Spigots
❑ Outside water spigots protected by hose bibb vacuum breakers

❑ Outside water spigots not protected by hose bibb vacuum breakers

Building Systems 65. Chimney and Exhaust Ventilation for Fuel-fired Equipment
❑ Improper exhaust venting: Any misalignment, blockage, rust, corrosion, or other deficiency that may cause improper or dangerous venting of exhaust gases
-OR-There is no pressure relief valve

❑ Proper exhaust venting: flue ok

❑ No chimney exhaust ventilation system required (e.g., electric water heater)

Building Systems 66. Makeup Air
❑ Makeup air not provided to the fireplace, gas water heater, or other fuel-burning fixtures

❑ Makeup air provided to the fireplace, gas water heater, or other fuel-burning fixtures

ELECTRICAL SYSTEMS
Building Systems 67. Breakers/Fuses
❑ Damaged breakers or fuses, frayed wiring, arcing scars: Carbon residue, melted breakers, or arcing scars

❑ Missing breakers/open panels/missing covers: Missing breakers or open panels (breaker port or receptacle or panel cover)

❑ Improper fusing: Fuse receptacles with improper fuses or bypassed

❑ Access blocked; could not inspect: The electrical system could not be visually accessed because of blockage or inaccessibility

❑ No deficiency observed

NOTE: Do not attempt to disassemble any electrical component or touch any circuit.

Building Systems 68. Water Leaks or Corrosion On or Near Electrical Systems

❑Evidence of water leaks/corrosion: Any corrosion that affects the condition of the components that carry current

-OR-Any stains or rust on the interior of electrical enclosures

-OR-Any evidence of water leaks in the enclosure or hardware

❑No evidence of water leaks/corrosion

Building Systems 69. Wiring

❑Deteriorated insulation exposing conducting wire: Nicks, abrasions, or fraying of the insulation exposing any conducting wire. **Do not check this for a bare grounding wire.**

❑No deteriorated insulation

Building Systems 70. Extension Cord Use

❑Extension cords not used properly: Extension cords under carpets or across doorways

-OR-Too many appliances plugged into one extension cord

❑Extension cords used properly: Extension cords not draped across doorways or under carpets and not overloaded with too many appliances

❑No extension cord use

Building Systems 71. Extension Cord Condition

❑Not good: Extension cords cracked or frayed

❑Good: Extension cords not cracked or frayed

❑No extension cord use

Building Systems 72. Electrical Covers

❑One or more missing covers: A cover is missing, which results in exposed visible electrical connections

❑Covers not missing

FIRE PROTECTION

Building Systems 73. Fire Sprinklers

❑Sprinkler disabled, missing, blocked, or painted over: Any sprinkler head is missing, visibly disabled, painted over, blocked, capped or otherwise disabled. **REPORT TO BUILDING MANAGEMENT/ OWNER IMMEDIATELY AND RECORD SPECIFICS IN THE COMMENTS SECTION.**

❑No sprinkler system

❑Sprinkler not disabled/missing/blocked

Building Systems 74. Missing, Damaged, Expired, or Wrong Kind of Fire Extinguishers/Fire Hoses

❑**≥10%, or none in building:** More than 10% of the fire extinguishers are missing, damaged, or expired. **IF THERE ARE NO FIRE EXTINGUISHERS, REPORT TO BUILDING MANAGEMENT/ OWNER IMMEDIATELY AND RECORD SPECIFICS IN THE COMMENTS SECTION.**
-OR-There is not an operable/non-expired fire extinguisher on each floor
-OR-The building does not have a fire extinguisher

❑**≥5% to <10%:** 5%–10% of the fire extinguishers are missing, damaged, expired, or wrong kind

❑**<1% to <5%:** <1% to <5% of extinguishers missing/damaged/expired or wrong kind

❑None missing/damaged/expired

Building Systems 75. Emergency Exit/Egress Routes

❑**All exits not clear of furniture, toys, and clutter**

❑All exits clear of furniture, toys, and clutter

HVAC

Building Systems 76. Boiler/Pump

❑**Water or steam leaks:** Water or steam leaking in piping or pump packing or boiler

❑No leaks

❑Does not apply

NOTE: This does not include fuel supply leaks, which are addressed in Building Systems 77.

Building Systems 77. Fuel Supply

❑**Leaks observed or odor of natural gas, propane, or oil detected:** Any amount of fuel is leaking from the supply tank or piping. **REPORT LEAKS TO BUILDING MANAGEMENT/OWNER IMMEDIATELY AND RECORD SPECIFICS IN THE COMMENTS SECTION. THE ODOR OF NATURAL GAS OR PROPANE IS AN IMMINENT HEALTH HAZARD; THE STRUCTURE SHOULD BE EVACUATED.**

❑No leaks observed or odor detected

❑Does not apply

Building Systems 78. Chimney Exhaust

❑Reversed air flow in chimney observed. **REPORT TO BUILDING MANAGEMENT/OWNER IMMEDIATELY AND RECORD SPECIFICS IN THE COMMENTS SECTION.**

❑**Misaligned, damaged, blocked, or disconnected:** Misalignment of an exhaust system on a gas-fired or oil-fired unit that causes improper or dangerous venting of gases
-OR-Evidence of blockage or disconnection
-OR-Evidence of rust and corrosion that could cause improper flue pipe and chimney function

❑Not misaligned, damaged, blocked, or disconnected

❑No chimney exhaust ventilation required

Building Systems 79. Chimney Spark Arrestor and Rain Cap

❏No chimney spark arrestor or rain cap

❏Chimney spark arrestor and rain cap installed

❏No chimney

Building Systems 80. HVAC Condensate and Sewage Corrosion

❏**Rust or corrosion prevents functioning:** Significant formations of metal oxides, significant flaking, discoloration, or the development of a noticeable pit or crevice
-OR-Equipment or piping does not function because of this condition
-OR-A drain is clogged or components of the sanitary system are leaking.
-OR-Evidence of standing water, puddles, or ponding (a sign of leaks or clogged drains)

❏**Some rust or corrosion or other damage, but system functioning**

❏No rust/corrosion

❏Not applicable: No ducts or pipes

Building Systems 81. HVAC Air Supply

❏**From basement only**

❏**Supply (return) air entirely from living area**

❏Supply (return) air includes fresh (outdoor) air

❏No forced air system present

COMMON AREAS (ITEMS 82–102)

NOTE: This section is for multihome sites only. If this is a single-family home, skip to Item 103.

Items to inspect in this category include
- Walkways/steps
- Ceilings
- Floors

A comment area for the common areas category is also included in this section.

ELEVATORS
Common Areas 82. Elevators
- ❏ Elevators and elevator equipment do not work properly
- ❏ Elevators and elevator equipment work properly
- ❏ No elevators

SIGNAGE
Common Areas 83. Exit Signage
- ❏ Exit signs missing or broken or not visible
- ❏ Exit signs present and functioning

SMOKING AREA
Common Areas 84. Designated Smoking Area
- ❏ Area littered with butts/food debris
- ❏ No butts/food debris observed
- ❏ No designated smoking area

INTERIOR TRASH
Common Areas 85. Trash Collection Areas
- ❏ **Trash on floor:** Extensive trash and/or garbage on the floor
- ❏ **Trash containers/chutes missing covers:** Missing or damaged covers to trash chutes or trash or garbage containers
- ❏ **Both:** Both trash on floor and missing or damaged covers
- ❏ No trash on floor or missing covers

OUTLETS, SWITCHES, COVER PLATES
Common Areas 86. Electrical Outlets
- ❏ Exposed wiring
- ❏ Missing cover plates
- ❏ **Both:** Both exposed wiring and missing cover plates
- ❏ No exposed wiring or missing cover plates

SMOKE AND CARBON MONOXIDE DETECTORS

Common Areas 87. Smoke Detectors

❑**Not operational:** One smoke detector tested per inspected common area; detector does not work as designed

❑**No smoke detector:** No smoke detectors in common area

❑**Operational:** One smoke detector tested per inspected common area; detector works as designed

NOTE: Test one per inspected common area if feasible.

Common Areas 88. Carbon Monoxide Detectors

❑**Not operational:** One CO detector tested per inspected common area; detector does not work as designed

❑**No carbon monoxide detector:** No CO detectors in common area

❑**Operational:** One CO detector tested per inspected common area; detector works as designed

NOTE: Test one per inspected common area if feasible.

WALKWAYS/STEPS

Common Areas 89. Walkways/Steps

❑**Missing/damaged/loose:** Walkways and steps have missing surfaces or are otherwise damaged
-OR-A missing or loose handrailing

❑No damage

❑No walkway/steps

CEILING

Common Areas 90. Ceiling Buckling

❑**Bulging or buckling:** Bulging, buckling, sagging, or a lack of horizontal alignment

❑No bulging/buckling

Common Areas 91. Ceiling Holes

❑**Large holes:** Total area larger than 8½ inches × 11 inches
-OR-A hole penetrates the area above
-OR-More than three tiles or panels are missing

❑**Small holes:** Total area not larger than 8½ inches × 11 inches
-OR-No hole penetrates the area above
-OR-No more than three tiles or panels are missing

❑No holes observed

Common Areas 92. Peeling/Needs Paint

❑**≥2 square feet:** More than 2 square feet of peeling or deteriorated paint in one or more common areas

❑**<2 square feet:** Less than 2 square feet of peeling or deteriorated paint in one or more common areas

❑**All intact:** All paint intact

Common Areas 93. Water Stains/Water Damage

❏**≥2 square feet:** One or more ceilings(s) has evidence of a leak, water damage, or water staining (such as a darkened area) over a large area (more than 4 square feet)

❏**<2 square feet:** One or more ceiling(s) has evidence of a leak, water damage, or water staining (such as a darkened area) over a small area (less than 4 square feet)

❏No water stains/water damage

NOTE: This does not include visible mold on ceiling, which is addressed in Common Areas 94.

Common Areas 94. Mold

❏**≥4 square feet mold observed or musty odor detected:** On one or more ceilings(s), mold is seen in a large area (more than 4 square feet) or there is a musty odor

❏**<4 square feet visible mold:** On one or more ceiling(s), mold is seen in a small area (less than 4 square feet)

❏No mold or musty odor

NOTE: This does not include water stains or damage on ceiling, which is addressed in Common Areas 93.

Common Areas 95. Mold Source

❏Leaking roof

❏Leaking appliance

❏Leaking water pipe in wall or ceiling

❏Poor ventilation

❏Do not know

FLOORS

Common Areas 96. Floor Buckling

❏**Yes:** Bulging, buckling, sagging, or alignment problem

❏No: Bulging, buckling, sagging, or alignment problem

Common Areas 97. Floor Covering

❏**≥50% damaged:** For one or more floor(s), more than 50% of the floor covering is damaged -OR-Damage to the floor covering exposes the underlying material

❏**10%–<50% damaged:** An estimated 10%–50% of the floor covering has stains, surface burns, shallow cuts, small holes, tears, loose areas, exposed seams, or other defect. The covering is fully functional, and there is no safety hazard.

❏**<10% damaged:** Less than 10% of the floor covering has stains, surface burns, shallow cuts, small holes, tears, loose areas, exposed seams, or other defect. The covering is fully functional, and there is no safety hazard.

❏No damage observed on any of the floors

Common Areas 98. Flooring/Tiles

❑≥50% missing or damaged: More than 50% of the flooring is affected by small holes and damage. -OR-The condition causes a safety problem

❑10%–<50% missing or damaged: An estimated 10%–50% of the flooring has small holes in areas of the floor surface, but there are no safety problems

❑<10% missing or damaged: For a single floor, there are small holes in areas of the floor surface. Less than 10% of the floor is affected and there are no safety problems.

❑No damaged or missing flooring

Common Areas 99. Peeling or Deteriorated Paint

❑≥2 square feet: Peeling or deteriorated paint in an area larger than 2 square feet in any one room or common area

❑<2 square feet: Peeling or deteriorated paint in an area smaller than 2 square feet in any one room or common area

❑No peeling or deteriorated paint

Common Areas 100. Subfloor

❑≥4 square feet rotting or deteriorated: Large areas of rot (more than 4 square feet) seen -OR-Applying weight to the floor causes noticeable deflection

❑<4 square feet rotting or deteriorated

❑Subfloor cannot be observed

Common Areas 101. Waters Stains/Water Damage

❑≥4 square feet: A large portion of one of more floors (more than 4 square feet) has been substantially saturated or damaged by water, mold, or mildew. Cracks, mold, and flaking are seen; the floor surface may have failed.

❑<4 square feet: Evidence of a water stain (such as a darkened area) over a small area of floor (less than 4 square feet). Water may or may not be seen. Less than 10% of the floors are affected.

❑No water stains/water damage

NOTE: This does not include visible mold on floor, which is addressed in Common Areas 102.

Common Areas 102. Mold

❑≥4 square feet mold observed or musty odor detected: On one or more floor(s) there is evidence of mold over a large area (more than 4 square feet) -OR-A musty odor is detected

❑<4 square feet visible mold: On one or more floor(s) there is evidence of mold over a small area (less than 4 square feet)

❑No visible mold present

NOTE: This does not include water stains or damage on floor, which is addressed in Common Areas 101.

HOUSING UNIT (ITEMS 103–196)

Items to inspect in this area are

- Bathroom
- Ceiling, floors, and walls
- Doors
- Electrical
- Water heater
- HVAC system
- Kitchen
- Laundry area
- Lighting
- Patio/porch/deck/balcony
- Smoke and carbon monoxide detectors
- Stairs
- Windows

A comment area for the housing unit category is included in this section.

BATHROOM

Housing Unit 103. Bathroom Cabinets

❏**Damaged:** Shelves, vanity tops, or drawers damaged or doors not functioning as they should

❏**Missing:** Shelves, vanity tops, drawers, or doors missing

❏**Both:** Both damaged and missing elements seen

❏No damage/missing cabinets

Housing Unit 104. Lavatory Sink

❏**≥50% discoloration or cracks:** The sink cannot be used because of extensive discoloration or cracks
   -OR-The sink or associated hardware is missing or has failed

❏**<50% discoloration or cracks:** The sink can be used, but there are either cracks or extensive discoloration affecting less than 50% of the basin
   -OR-A stopper is missing

❏No cracks/discoloration

NOTE: This does not include clogged drains, which are addressed in Housing Unit 105.

Housing Unit 105. Plumbing Drain

❏**Drain completely clogged:** Fixtures are not usable because the drain is completely clogged or shows extensive deterioration

❏**Slow drain:** Water does not drain freely, but the fixtures can be used

❏Drain working properly

Housing Unit 106. Plumbing Faucets/Fixtures

❑**Large water leak:** There is a steady leak adversely affecting the area around it
   -OR-The faucet or pipe cannot be used

❑**Small water leak:** There is a leak or drip contained by the basin

❑No leaks observed

Housing Unit 107. Water Temperature

❑**Only hot water present,** but not hotter than 120°F

❑**Only cold water present**

❑Hot and cold water present

Housing Unit 108. Water Pressure

❑**Inadequate at any bathroom plumbing fixtures**

❑Adequate at all bathroom plumbing fixtures

Housing Unit 109. Shower/Tub Surface

❑**≥50% or surface area damaged, inoperable or missing:** The shower or tub can be used but there are cracks or extensive discoloration in more than 50% of the basin surface area
   -OR-The shower or tub cannot be used for any reason
   -OR-The shower, tub, faucets, drains, or associated hardware are missing or have failed

❑**<50% of surface area damaged:** The shower or tub can be used but there are cracks or extensive discoloration in less than 50% of the surface area of the basin or stall

❑No damage

NOTE: This does not include leaking faucets or pipes, which are addressed in Housing Unit 106.

Housing Unit 110. Shower/Tub Grab Bars

❑Grab bars not installed

❑Grab bars improperly installed

❑Grab bars properly installed inside and outside of tub

NOTE: Applies to households with elderly residents or a resident with a physical handicap.

Housing Unit 111. Bathroom Exhaust

❑**Exhaust fan not working**
   -OR-No exhaust fan or window present

❑Exhaust fan working

Housing Unit 112. Toilet

❏Toilet seat and/or bowl cracked or broken: Fixture elements (seat, flush handle, cover, etc.) are missing or damaged
-OR-There is a hazardous condition: **REPORT TO BUILDING MANAGEMENT/OWNER IMMEDIATELY AND RECORD SPECIFICS IN THE COMMENTS SECTION**
-OR-The bowl is fractured or broken and cannot retain water
-OR-The water closet/toilet is missing
-OR-The water closet/toilet cannot be flushed because of obstruction or another defect

❏Toilet seat cracked or broken

❏Not cracked or broken: A water closet/toilet is not damaged and functions properly

Housing Unit 113. Toilet Grab Bars

❏Grab bars not installed

❏Grab bars improperly installed

❏Grab bars properly installed next to toilet

NOTE: Applies to households with elderly residents or a resident with a physical handicap.

Housing Unit 114. Shower/Bath/Toilet Caulking and/or Seals

❏Deteriorated caulk/seals

❏No deterioration observed

Housing Unit 115. Bathroom Call-for-Aid

❏Damaged or not working

❏Missing

❏No call-for-aid unit

❏No damage/working/not missing

NOTE: Applies to households with elderly residents or a resident with a physical handicap.

Housing Unit 116. Permanent Carpet on Bathroom Floor

❏Permanent carpet: Does not include removable bath mats

❏No permanent carpet: Bathroom floor is a hard, cleanable surface

CEILING, FLOORS, AND WALLS
Housing Unit 117. Bulging/Buckling

❏Bulging, buckling, or alignment problem: Bulging, buckling, sagging, or alignment problem.

❏No bulging, buckling, or alignment problem

Housing Unit 118. Holes

❏**Large holes ≥8½ inches × 11 inches:** A hole is larger 8½ inches by 11 inches but it does not penetrate the area above or adjacent
-OR-More than three tiles or panels are missing
-OR-There is a crack more than ⅛ inch wide and 11 inches long
-OR-A hole penetrates the area above or adjacent

❏**Medium-sized holes present:** Holes less than 8½ inches × 11 inches in area
-OR-No hole penetrates the area above or adjacent
-OR-No more than three tiles or panels are missing

❏**Small holes present:** Holes smaller than 8½ inches × ½ inches (do not count pinholes) in total hole area.

❏No holes observed

Housing Unit 119. Peeling/Needs Paint

❏**≥2 square feet damage:** Peeling or deteriorated paint in an area larger than 2 square feet in any one room

❏**<2 square feet damage:** Peeling or deteriorated paint in an area smaller than 2 square feet in any one room

❏No damage/peeling paint

Housing Unit 120. Water Stains/Water Damage

❏**≥4 square feet water stains/water damage:** Any one ceiling, floor, or wall has evidence of water stains/water damage, a leak (such as a darkened area) over a large area (4 square feet or more). Water may or may not be visible.

❏**<4 square feet water stains/water damage:** Any one ceiling, floor, or wall has evidence of water stains/water damage, a leak (such as a darkened area) over a small area (less than 4 square feet). Water may or may not be visible.

❏No water stains/water damage

NOTE: This does not include visible mold, which is addressed in Housing Unit 122.

Housing Unit 121. Condensation on Windows

❏Condensation on windows, doors, walls

❏No condensation on windows, doors, walls

Housing Unit 122. Mold

❏**≥4 square feet visible mold present or musty odor detected:** Any one ceiling, floor, or wall has visible mold over a large area (4 square feet or more)
-OR-A musty odor is detected

❏**<4 square feet visible mold present:** Any one ceiling, floor, or wall has visible mold over a small area (less than 4 square feet)

❏No mold observed or musty odor detected

NOTE: This does not include water stains or damage, which are addressed in Housing Unit 120.

Housing Unit 123. Mold Source

❑Leaking roof

❑Leaking appliance

❑Leaking water pipe in wall or ceiling

❑Poor ventilation

❑Do not know

DOORS
Housing Unit 124. Door Surface

❑≥1 inch: One door has a hole or holes equal to or larger than 1 inch in diameter in total surface area, significant peeling/cracking/no paint, rust that affects the integrity of the door surface, or broken/missing glass

❑¼ inch to 1 inch diameter: One interior door—not a bathroom or entry door—has a hole or holes or peeling cracking no paint, or rust with a diameter ranging from ¼ inch to 1 inch in total surface area

❑No damaged surface observed
124b. If door surface(s) are damaged, record door location _____

Housing Unit 125. Frame/Threshold/Lintel/Trim

❑Bathroom or entry door not working (closing, opening and/or latching): At least one bathroom door or entry door is not functioning or cannot be locked because of damage to the frame, threshold, lintel, or trim or door hardware

❑At least one interior door not working (closing, opening and/or latching): At least one door is not functioning or cannot be locked because of damage to the frame, threshold, lintel, or trim or hardware

❑Both: Both bathroom or entry door and other interior door not working

❑No damage observed: All doors functioning

Housing Unit 126. Seals (Entry Only)

❑Entry door seals deteriorated/missing: The seals are missing on one or more entry door(s), or they are so damaged that they do not function as they should

❑No damage observed

Housing Unit 127. Door Missing

❑Bathroom door missing

❑One or more missing (not bathroom or entry): A door is missing, but it is not a bathroom door or entry door

❑Entry door missing

❑None missing

Housing Unit 128. Deadbolt Locks

❏Deadbolt locks cannot be unlocked from the inside without a key

❏No deadbolt locks

❏Deadbolt locks can be unlocked from the inside without a key

Housing Unit 129. Door Lock Operation

❏Door locks cannot be operated by a child in an emergency

❏No door locks

❏Door locks can be operated by a child in an emergency

ELECTRICAL

Housing Unit 130. Electrical Panel Access

❏Yes: One or more fixed items or items of sufficient size and weight can impede access to the unit's electrical panel during an emergency

❏No: Access is not impeded

Housing Unit 131. Breakers/Fuses

❏**Damaged breakers or fuses, frayed wiring, arcing scars:** Carbon residue, melted breakers, or arcing scars

❏**Missing breakers/open panels/missing covers:** Missing breakers or open panels (breaker port or receptacle or panel cover)

❏**Improper fusing:** Fuse receptacles with improper or bypassed fuses

❏**Access blocked; could not inspect:** Electrical system could not be visually accessed due to blockage or inaccessibility

❏No deficiency observed

NOTE: Do not attempt to disassemble any electrical component or touch any circuit.

Housing Unit 132. Water Leaks or Corrosion Near Electrical Systems

❏Yes: Any leaks or corrosion
    -OR-Any stains or rust on the interior of electrical enclosures
    -OR-Any evidence of water leaks in the enclosure or any hardware deficiency (such as nicks, abrasions, or fraying of the insulation that expose wires that conduct current). **NOTE:** Do not consider this a deficiency for wires that are not intended to be insulated, such as grounding wires.

❏No: Leaks or corrosion not observed

Housing Unit 133. Wiring

❏**Deteriorated electrical insulation:** Nicks, abrasions, or fraying of the insulation that exposes any conducting wire

❏No deterioration

Housing Unit 134. Ground Fault Circuit Interrupters (GFCI)
❏Inoperable or missing

❏Operable

Housing Unit 135. Arc Fault Circuit Interrupters (AFCI)
❏Inoperable or missing

❏Operable

Housing Unit 136. Missing or Broken Electrical Covers
❏**Exposed wiring:** An open breaker port or exposed wiring
   -OR-A cover is missing and electrical connections are exposed

❏None missing/broken/exposed

Housing Unit 137. Child Tamper-resistant Outlet Covers
❏**No tamper-resistant outlet covers in units with young children**

❏Installed tamper-resistant outlet covers in units with young children

❏Not applicable (no young children in unit)

Housing Unit 138. Extension Cord Use
❏**Extension cords not used properly:** Extension cords under carpets or across doorways
   -OR-Too many appliances plugged into one extension cord

❏Extension cords used properly: Extension cords not draped across doorways or under carpets and not
   overloaded with too many appliances

❏No extension cord use

Housing Unit 139. Extension Cord Condition
❏**Not good:** Extension cords cracked or frayed

❏Good: Extension cords not cracked or frayed

❏No extension cord use

WATER HEATER
Housing Unit 140. Water Heater Exhaust
❏**Misaligned:** Any misalignment that may cause improper or dangerous venting of gases.

❏Not misaligned

❏Does not apply: Electrical hot water or heater used instead of gas-fired or oil-fired unit
   -OR-No water heater inside unit.

NOTE: If no water heater inside unit, skip to question 145.

Housing Unit 141. Water Temperature

❏Temperature set at or above 120°F

❏No hot water

❏Temperature set below 120°F

Housing Unit 142. Leaks

❏Water leak observed

❏No water leak observed

Housing Unit 143. Water Heater Temperature/Pressure Relief Valve

❏Absent

❏Present

NOTE: Do not operate the relief valve.

Housing Unit 144. Water Heater Secured

❏Not strapped down

❏Strapped down

HVAC SYSTEM

Housing Unit 145. General Rust/Corrosion (HVAC)

❏**Significant rust/corrosion:** Significant deterioration from rust and corrosion on HVAC units in the dwelling unit (includes ducts, radiators, baseboard heaters, etc.). The system does not provide sufficient heating or cooling.

❏**Surface rust/corrosion:** Deterioration from rust and corrosion on HVAC units in the dwelling unit (includes ducts, radiators, baseboard heaters, etc.). The system still provides sufficient heating or cooling.

❏No rust/corrosion in HVAC units in the dwelling unit (includes ducts, radiators, baseboard heaters, etc.)

Housing Unit 146. HVAC Operation

❏**Not working:** HVAC system does not function; it does not provide the heating or cooling it should. The system does not respond when the controls are engaged.

❏Working

Housing Unit 147. Supply Air for HVAC (From Basement Only)

❏Supply (return) air entirely from living area

❏No forced air system present

❏Supply (return) air includes fresh (outdoor) air

Housing Unit 148. HVAC Filters

❏Need replacement

❏Clean

❏Not applicable

Housing Unit 149. HVAC Exhaust Ventilation System

☐Reversed air flow in chimney observed: **REPORT TO BUILDING MANAGEMENT/OWNER IMMEDIATELY AND RECORD SPECIFICS IN THE COMMENTS SECTION**

☐Misaligned, damaged, blocked, rusted, corroded, or disconnected

☐Not misaligned, damaged, blocked, or disconnected

☐No exhaust ventilation required (e.g., electric or no HVAC systems in unit)

Housing Unit 150. HVAC Noise

☐Noisy/vibrating/leaking: HVAC system shows signs of abnormal vibrations, other noise, or leaks when engaged

☐Not noisy

☐Does not apply: No HVAC inside unit

Housing Unit 151. Space Heaters

☐Space heaters used in unit are not at least 3 feet from anything that can burn

☐Space heaters used in unit are at least 3 feet from anything that can burn

☐Not applicable: No space heaters used in unit

Housing Unit 152. Fireplace Screen

☐Fireplace does not have a sturdy screen to catch sparks

☐Fireplace has a sturdy screen to catch sparks

☐Not applicable: No fireplace in unit

Housing Unit 153. Fireplace Dampers

☐Fireplace dampers not operational

☐Fireplace dampers operational

☐Not applicable: No fireplace in unit

Housing Unit 154. Wood Stove Barrier

☐No barrier to keep children from getting too close to wood stove surfaces

☐Barrier in place to keep children away from wood stove surfaces

☐Not applicable: No wood stove in unit

KITCHEN

Housing Unit 155. Cabinets

☐≥50% cabinets or cabinet doors missing: More than 50% of the cabinets or doors are missing

☐<50% cabinets or cabinet doors missing: Less than 50% of the cabinets, doors, or shelves are missing

☐No doors missing

Housing Unit 156. Cabinet Damage

☐≥20% damaged or laminate separation

☐<20% damaged or laminate separation

☐No damage or laminate separation

Housing Unit 157. Countertops

☐≥20% missing/damaged: More than 20% of the countertop working surface is missing, deteriorated, or damaged below the laminate. Countertop is not a sanitary surface on which to prepare food.

☐<20% missing/damaged: 20% or less of the countertop working surface is missing, deteriorated, or damaged below the laminate. Countertop is not a sanitary surface on which to prepare food.

☐No missing/damaged countertops

Housing Unit 158. Dishwasher

☐Not working: The dishwasher does not function as it should

☐Working

☐No dishwasher

Housing Unit 159. Garbage Disposal

☐Not working: The garbage disposal does not function as it should

☐Working

☐No garbage disposal

Housing Unit 160. Kitchen Drain

☐Kitchen drain completely clogged: Drain completely clogged or extensively deteriorated

☐Slow kitchen drain: Basin does not drain freely

☐Kitchen drain working properly

Housing Unit 161. Kitchen Plumbing

☐Steady leak/adverse effect: A steady leak is having an adverse affect on the surrounding area -OR-The kitchen faucet or pipe is not usable

☐Leak contained by kitchen sink: A leak or drip is contained by the basin or pipes and the faucet is functioning properly

☐No leak

Housing Unit 162. Electrical
    ❑No GFCI near kitchen sink
      -OR-GFCI does not work properly

    ❑GFCI is near kitchen sink and it works properly

Housing Unit 163. Water Temperature
    ❑Only hot water present at kitchen plumbing fixtures

    ❑Only cold water present at kitchen plumbing fixtures

    ❑Hot and cold water present at kitchen plumbing fixtures

Housing Unit 164. Water Pressure
    ❑Inadequate water pressure at kitchen plumbing fixtures

    ❑Adequate water pressure at all kitchen plumbing fixtures

Housing Unit 165. Range Hood
    ❑**Not working:** Range hood does not turn on

    ❑**Partial blockage:** An accumulation of dirt threatens the free passage of air
      -OR-Flue completely blocked

    ❑No range hood/exhaust fan

    ❑No blockage/functional: Range hood works properly

Housing Unit 166. Range or Stove
    ❑Stove and/or oven missing

    ❑**Two or more burners not working**
      Gas ranges: flames not distributed equally or pilot lights out on two or more burners
      Electric ranges: two or more heating elements (including the oven) not working

    ❑**One burner not working:**
      Gas ranges: flames not distributed equally or pilot lights out on one burner
      Electric ranges: one heating element (including the oven) not working

    ❑Stove and oven working

Housing Unit 167. Refrigerator
    ❑Refrigerator missing or inoperable

    ❑**Seals deteriorated:** Refrigerator has an excessive accumulation of ice
      -OR-Seals around refrigerator doors are deteriorated
      -OR-Refrigerator does not cool adequately for the safe food storage (temperature above 40°F)

    ❑Refrigerator functioning properly (temperature 40°F or below)

Housing Unit 168. Kitchen Sink

❑**≥50% discoloration, chips, or cracks or inoperable:** Sink cannot be used because of extensive discoloration, chips, or cracks
-OR-Sink cannot be used because the sink or associated hardware is missing or has failed

❑**<50% discoloration, chips, or cracks:** Sink can be used but cracks, chips, or extensive discoloration are seen in less than 50% of the basin
-OR-A stopper is missing

❑No cracks/discoloration/chips; sink operable

Housing Unit 169. Permanent Carpet on Kitchen Floor

❑**Permanent carpet on kitchen floor** (does not include removable mats)

❑Kitchen floor is a hard, cleanable surface

Housing Unit 170. Cleaning Products

❑**Cleaning products not stored out of the reach of children**

❑Cleaning products stored out of the reach of children

❑No cleaning products stored in kitchen area

LAUNDRY AREA

Housing Unit 171. Clothes Dryer

❑**Vent missing:** Dryer vent to outside is missing

❑**Vent damaged:** Dryer exhaust is not effectively vented to the outside because of blockage or inadequate design or is vented into the interior

❑Vent not missing or damaged: Exhaust vent is functioning properly

❑No dryer

Housing Unit 172. Exhaust Duct From Dryer

❑**Flexible plastic:** Dryer exhaust duct is made of flexible plastic

❑**Flexible metal:** Dryer exhaust duct is made of flexible metal

❑Other: Wood or other combustible material

❑Rigid metal: Dryer exhaust duct is made of rigid metal

Housing Unit 173. Dryer Venting

❑Dryer vents to basement

❑Dryer vents to attic

❑Dryer vents to crawl space

❑Other: _____

❑Dryer vents to outside

LIGHTING

Housing Unit 174. Interior Housing Unit Lighting

❏**One or more lights missing:** In one or more rooms in a unit, a permanent lighting fixture is missing, and no other switched light source is functioning in the room

❏**One or more lights not working:** In one or more rooms in a unit, a permanent lighting fixture is not working, and no other switched light source is functioning in the room

❏All lights working/none missing

Housing Unit 175. Outlets/Switches

❏**Broken, wires exposed:** Broken cover plates with wires exposed
-OR-Outlets or switches missing

❏**Broken, but no exposed wires**

❏No broken cover plates

PATIO/PORCH/DECK/BALCONY

Housing Unit 176. Railings

❏**Missing:** The baluster or side rails are missing

❏**Loose or damaged:** The baluster or side rails enclosing this area are loose or damaged

❏No damage

Housing Unit 177. Electrical Outlets

❏**No GFCIs present**
-OR-**GFCIs not functional**

❏GFCIs present and functional

❏No exterior outlets

Housing Unit 178. Spindles and Railings

❏**Missing:** Spindles or railings missing on porch, deck, or balcony

❏**Present:** Spindles and railings present on porch, deck, or balcony

❏Not applicable: No porch, deck, or balcony

Housing Unit 179. Spindles and Railings: Condition

❏Damaged

❏Loose

❏Too low

❏Too far apart

❏Missing

❏Good condition and properly spaced

❏Not applicable: No porch, deck, or balcony

Housing Unit 180. Spindles

❑Spindles more than 4 inches apart

❑Spindles not more than 4 inches apart

❑Not applicable: No porch, deck, or balcony

Housing Unit 181. Railing Height

❑Railing is not between 30 and 42 inches in height

❑Railing is between 30 and 42 inches in height

❑Not applicable: No porch, deck, or balcony

Housing Unit 182. Patio Surface

❑≥¾ inch displacement

❑≤¾ inch displacement

❑Uneven steps

❑No cracks/level

SMOKE AND CARBON MONOXIDE DETECTORS

Housing Unit 183. Smoke Detectors

❑Not operational: At least one smoke detector tested in each unit; detector does not work as designed

❑No smoke detector present: No smoke detector in unit

❑Operational: One smoke detector tested in each unit (if feasible); detector works as designed

Housing Unit 184. Smoke Detector Location

❑No smoke detectors in unit

❑Smoke detectors in home, but not on every level, outside each bedroom, and in a common living area

❑Smoke detectors on every level of the home, outside each bedroom, and in a common living area

Housing Unit 185. Smoke Detector Power

❑No smoke detectors in unit

❑Smoke detector powered by main electrical supply without battery backup

❑Smoke detector powered by battery

❑Smoke detector powered by main electrical supply with battery backup

Housing Unit 186. CO Detectors

❑Not operational: At least one CO detector tested in each unit; detector does not work as designed

❑No CO detector present: No CO detector in unit

❑Operational: All CO detectors tested in each unit (if feasible); all detector(s) work as designed

Housing Unit 187. CO Detector Location

❏No CO detectors in unit

❏CO detector in dwelling unit but not near bedroom area

❏CO detector near bedroom area

Housing Unit 188. Fire Extinguisher

❏No fire extinguisher present

❏Fire extinguisher present in home

❏Fire extinguisher present in home and charged

STAIRS

Housing Unit 189. Stair Railings

❏**Missing:** Handrail missing

❏**Broken, insecure, or missing:** Handrail damaged, loose, or otherwise unusable or insecure

❏Handrail present on both sides and not broken, missing, or insecure

❏Does not apply: No stairs or three or fewer stairs

Housing Unit 190. Steps: Condition

❏**One or more broken or missing:** One or more steps are broken or missing

❏Not broken or missing: No broken or missing steps

❏Does not apply: No steps

Housing Unit 191. Steps: Covering

❏No covering on stairs

❏Covering on stairs is not firmly attached or is poor condition

❏Covering on stairs (e.g., nonslip tread covers) is firmly attached and in good condition

WINDOWS

Housing Unit 192. Windows

❏One or more windows missing

❏One or more windows cracked or broken

❏One or more windows cannot be opened

❏All windows intact and can be opened

Housing Unit 193. Window Sills

❑**Missing or damaged:** A sill is missing or damaged, but the inside of the surrounding wall is not exposed and is still weathertight

❑**Not weathertight:** A sill is missing or damaged enough to expose the inside of the surrounding wall and compromise its weather tightness

❑Not missing or damaged

Housing Unit 194. Window Locks

❑Not functioning and cannot be secured/locked

❑Not functioning but can be secured/locked

❑Functioning and lockable

Housing Unit 195. Window Caulking/Seals

❑**Missing/deteriorated (leaks present):** There is missing or deteriorated caulk or seals and evidence of leaks or damage to the window or surrounding structure

❑**Missing/deteriorated (no leaks):** There is missing or deteriorated caulk on widows, but there is no evidence of damage to the window or surrounding structure

❑Not missing/deteriorated

Housing Unit 196. Window Paint

❑**Deteriorating paint:** Deteriorating paint or a window that needs paint on 10% or more of its surface

❑**No deteriorating paint:** All paint intact or deteriorating paint on less than 10% of the surface

COMMENTS, HOUSING UNIT SECTION

OTHER ITEMS (ITEMS 197–229)

Issues to assess in this area include

- Garbage and debris
- Injury hazards
- Childproofing measures
- Poisoning hazards
- Pest hazards
- Moisture hazards
- Swimming pool, spa, or whirlpool
- Other hazards

A comment area for the other items category is also included in this section.

GARBAGE AND DEBRIS

Other 197. Indoors

❑**Garbage and debris not properly stored:** Missing, uncovered, or leaking container

❑Garbage and debris properly stored

NOTE: This does not include garbage or debris improperly stored outside, which are addressed in Other 198.

Other 198. Outdoors

❑**Garbage and debris not properly stored:** Missing, uncovered, or leaking container

❑Garbage and debris properly stored

NOTE: This does not include garbage or debris improperly stored inside, which are addressed in Other 197.

INJURY HAZARDS

Other 199. Sharp Edges

❑**Yes:** Physical hazard present that could produce a skin cut or injury

❑No: Sharp edges not present

199b. If yes, record location(s): _____

Other 200. Trip Hazards

❑**Yes:** Tripping hazards present

❑No: Tripping hazards not present

200b. If yes, record location(s): _____

Other 201. Garage Door Opener

❑**Garage door does not reverse properly**

❑Garage door opener reverses properly

❑No garage door or no garage

CHILDPROOFING MEASURES

NOTE: These questions pertain to households where young children live or visit. If young children do not live in or visit the house/unit, skip to Other 208.

Other 202. Window Cords (Strangulation Hazard)
    ❑**Yes:** Window cords looped or tied together

    ❑No: Window cords not looped or tied together

202b. If yes, record location: _____

Other 203. Window Guards
    ❑Missing or not operational

    ❑Present and operational

Other 204. Cabinet Locks
    ❑Childproof cabinet locks missing or not operational

    ❑Childproof cabinet locks in place and operational

Other 205. Water Safety
    ❑Toilets not covered (toilet lids open)

    ❑Toilets covered (toilet lids closed)

Other 206. Chemicals, Pesticides, Cleaning Supplies, or Medications Stored Within Easy Reach of Children
    ❑Yes

    ❑No
206b. If yes, record type and location: _____

Other 207. Hobbies
    ❑**Evidence of household hobbies that could pose a risk to young children**

    ❑No evidence of household hobbies that could pose a risk to young children

POISONING HAZARDS
Other 208. Unvented Combustion Appliances
    ❑**Yes:** Unvented combustion appliances (e.g., fuel-fired space heaters, gas clothes dryers, gas logs, charcoal, stoves etc.) present

    ❑No: Unvented combustion appliances (e.g., fuel-fired space heaters, gas clothes dryers, gas logs, charcoal, stoves etc.) not present
208b. If yes, record type and number: _____

Other 209. Attached Garage

❑Attached garage not sealed from living area

❑**Do not know:** Not sure whether attached garage sealed from living area

❑Attached garage sealed from living area

❑Not applicable: No attached garage

PEST HAZARDS

Other 210. Infestation: Roaches

❑Frass or shells

❑One or more live roaches

❑No roaches or roach evidence

210b. If roach evidence present, record location(s): _____

NOTE: This does not include infestations of other other pests, which are addressed in Other 211 and 212.

Other 211. Infestation: Rats or Mice

❑Droppings or chewed holes

❑One or more rats/mice

❑No rats/mice/droppings/holes

211b. If rat or mouse evidence present, record location(s): _____

NOTE: This does not include infestations of other pests, which are addressed in Other 210 (roaches) and Other 212 (other insects or vermin).

Other 212. Other Insects or Vermin

❑**Yes:** Other insects or vermin seen

❑No: Other insects or vermin not seen

212b. If yes, record and location(s) type: _____

Other 213. Termite Tunnels

❑**Yes:** Termite tunnels

❑No: No termite tunnels

213b. If seen, where in unit: _____

MOISTURE HAZARDS

Other 214. Sources of Excessive Humidity Present

❑Yes: Sources of humidity (e.g., humidifier, dryer vented inside, uncovered fish tank) present

❑No: Sources of humidity (e.g., humidifier, dryer vented inside, uncovered fish tank) not present

214b. If yes, record type and number: _____

Other 215. Moldy or Musty Odor Present

❑Yes

❑No

215b. If yes, record location: _____

Other 216. Dehumidifier Present

❑No

❑Yes

SWIMMING POOL, SPA, OR WHIRLPOOL

NOTE: These questions pertain to homes/units with a swimming pool, spa, or whirlpool. If there are no swimming pools, spas, or whirlpools, skip to Other 224.

Other 217. Fencing and Gates

❑Missing or broken fencing or gate

❑Damaged fencing or gate open

❑Pool surrounded by undamaged three-sided fencing (house acts as fourth side)

❑Pool surrounded by undamaged four-sided fencing

Other 218. Doors and Gates

❑All doors and gates to swimming pool and spa areas do not close and latch automatically

❑All doors and gates to swimming pool and spa areas close and latch automatically

Other 219. Latches

❑Latching devices are not at least 48 inches from the ground

❑Latching devices are not self-closing, self latching

❑Self-closing, self-latching devices are at least 48 inches from the ground

Other 220. Safety Equipment (Swimming Pool)

❑None

❑Life ring

❑Shepherd's hook

❑Both life ring and shepherd's hook

Other 221. GFCI

❑No GFCI in area

❑GFCI present but not working

❑GFCI present and working in area

Other 222. Drain Cover

❑Drain cover missing or broken: **SHUT DOWN POOL, SPA, OR WHIRLPOOL IMMEDIATELY AND REPORT TO BUILDING MANAGEMENT/OWNER. RECORD SPECIFICS IN THE COMMENTS SECTION.**

❑Drain cover in place and not broken

Other 223. Safety Cover

❑No safety cover on spa

❑Unlocked safety cover on spa

❑Locked safety cover on spa

OTHER HAZARDS

Other 224. Visible Dust on Surfaces

❑Heavy

❑Slight

❑No visible dust on surfaces

Other 225. Air Cleaning Device Present

❑Yes

❑No

Other 226. Ozone Generator Present

❑Yes

❑No

Other 227. Pets Present

❑Yes

❑No

227b. If yes, record type and number of pet(s): _____

Other 228. Tobacco Smoke or Odor Present

❑Yes

❑No

Other 229. Other Hazards

❏Yes

❏No

229b. If yes, record type and location: _____

COMMENTS, OTHER ITEMS SECTION

OVERALL COMMENTS ON THIS INSPECTION

Add any other comments related to this inspection here.

APPENDIX 1:
DESCRIPTION OF HEALTH AND SAFETY CONDITIONS IDENTIFIED ON THE VISUAL ASSESSMENT FORM

Adapted from the HUD Public Housing Assessment System (PHAS) and its Physical Assessment Subsystem (PASS) as well as from inspection protocols used by healthy homes grantees.

> This inspection protocol does not establish legal and/or complete compliance with local, state, federal or other applicable housing, building, health, safety or other applicable policies, codes, regulations, statutes and laws.

IPMC code provisions cross-referenced in this appendix are listed in Appendix 2: 2003 International Property Maintenance Code (2003 IPMC) Cross-References.

DATA DICTIONARY:
MAJOR VISUAL ASSESSMENT AREAS

SITE (ITEMS 1–29)

Items to inspect in this category are
- Fencing and Gates
- Grounds or Pavement
- Children's Play Areas
- Other

FENCING AND GATES

FENCE: A structure functioning as a boundary or barrier. An upright structure serving to enclose, divide or protect an area.

GATE: A structured opening in a fence for entrance or exit.

NOTE: This does not include swimming pool fences. Swimming pool fences are covered in Other Items/ Swimming Pool, Spa, or Whirlpool.

SITE 1. Damaged/Falling/Leaning/Deteriorated Paint
(2003 IPMC CROSS-REFERENCE: 302.7 ACCESSORY STRUCTURES)

DEFICIENCY: A fence or gate is rusted, deteriorated, or uprooted and may threaten security, health, or safety. If the fence has deteriorated paint in an area larger than 20 square feet and the property was built before 1978, record this as damaged but not functional.

NOTE: Gates for swimming pool fences are covered in Other Items/Swimming Pool, Spa, or Whirlpool.

SITE 2. Holes or Openings in Soil Below Fence
(2003 IPMC CROSS-REFERENCE: NONE)

DEFICIENCY: There is an opening or penetration in any fence or gate designed to keep intruders out or children in. Look for holes that could allow animals to enter or could threaten the safety of children. There is an opening/hole in soil beneath the fence.

NOTE: If the fence or gate is not designed to keep intruders out or children in (such as a rail fence), do not evaluate it for holes or openings.

GROUNDS OR PAVEMENT

SITE 3. Areas of Erosion
(2003 IPMC CROSS-REFERENCE: 302.2 GRADING AND DRAINAGE)

The improved land adjacent to or surrounding the housing and related structures. This does not include land not owned or under the control of the homeowner or housing provider.

DEFICIENCY: Natural processes—weathering, erosion, or gravity—or human processes have caused any of these conditions: collection or removal of surface material or sunken tracks, ruts, grooves, or depressions.

NOTES: This does not include detention/retention

basins or ponding on paved areas such as parking lots. Detention/retention basins are covered in Site 24: Storm Drainage. Ponding on paved areas is covered in Site 7: Cracks in Pavement. If there has been measurable precipitation (1/10 inch or more) during the previous 48 hours, consider its impact on the extent of the ponding. Determine that ponding has occurred only when there is clear evidence of a persistent or long-standing problem.

SITE 4. Overgrown Vegetation
(2003 IPMC CROSS-REFERENCE: 302.4 WEEDS)

DEFICIENCY: Plant life has spread to unacceptable areas or unintended surfaces or has grown in areas where it was not intended to grow.

SITE 5. Graffiti
(2003 IPMC CROSS-REFERENCE: 302.9 DEFACEMENT OF PROPERTY)

DEFICIENCY: Crude inscriptions or drawings are scratched, painted, or sprayed on a building surface, retaining wall, or fence that the public can see from 30 feet away.

NOTE: There is a difference between art forms and graffiti. Do not consider full wall murals and other art forms as graffiti.

SITE 6. Litter
(2003 IPMC CROSS-REFERENCE: 302.1 SANITATION)

DEFICIENCY: There is a disorderly accumulation of objects on the property—especially carelessly discarded trash.

SITE 7. Cracks in Pavement
(2003 IPMC CROSS-REFERENCE: 302.3 SIDEWALKS AND DRIVEWAYS)

An area for parking motorized vehicles begins at the curbside and includes all parking lots, driveways, or roads within the property lines that are under the control of the homeowner or housing provider.

DEFICIENCY: There are visible faults (longitudinal, lateral, alligator, etc.) in the pavement.

NOTE: Do not include small cracks on walkways.

Relief joints are there by design; do not consider them cracks. When observing traffic ability, consider the capacity to support people on foot, in wheelchairs, and using walkers—and the potential for problems and hazards. For parking lots only, note a deficiency if there are cracks on more than 5% of the parking spaces. For driveways/roads, note a deficiency if there are cracks on more than 5% of the driveways/roads.

CHILDREN'S PLAY AREAS

SITE 10. Equipment
(2003 IPMC CROSS-REFERENCE: NONE)

An outdoor area set aside for recreation or play, especially an area containing equipment such as seesaws and swings. Surfaces around playground equipment should have at least 12 inches of wood chips, mulch, sand, pea gravel, or mats made of safety-tested rubber or rubber-like materials.

DEFICIENCY: Playground equipment is dangerous or broken. **IF ANY EQUIPMENT POSES AN IMMEDIATE THREAT: REPORT TO BUILDING MANAGEMENT/OWNER IMMEDIATELY AND RECORD SPECIFICS IN THE COMMENTS SECTION**

NOTE: Except when safety is still a concern (sharp edges, dangerous leaning, etc.), do not evaluate equipment that the owner states has been withdrawn from service. For example, if the owner removed the net and hoop from a basketball backboard and the backboard poses no safety hazards, it is not a deficiency.

SITE 11. Paint Condition
(2003 IPMC CROSS-REFERENCE: NONE)

DEFICIENCY: Deteriorated paint on ≥50% of play area equipment surface.

SITE 12. Bare Soil
(2003 IPMC CROSS-REFERENCE: NONE)

The presence of large areas of bare soil in play areas can be a soil lead hazard. This is especially a concern near structures built before 1978 or near areas where older structures were demolished and new ones built on the site.

DEFICIENCY: More than 9 square feet of bare soil present in play area.

SITE 13. Injury-absorbent Surface Depth
(2003 IPMC CROSS-REFERENCE: NONE)

DEFICIENCY: Wood chips, mulch, sand, pea gravel, or safety-tested rubber or rubberlike materials are present at a depth of less than 12 inches.

NOTE: The depth of these materials varies by material as well as the equipment it is installed around. The Consumer Product Safety Commission's *Handbook for Public Playground Safety* (http://www.cpsc.gov/CPSCPUB/PUBS/325.pdf) provides more-detailed information for surfaces and equipment.

SITE 14. Deteriorated Injury-absorbent Surface
(2003 IPMC CROSS-REFERENCE: 302.2 GRADING AND DRAINAGE)

DEFICIENCY: Damage to a play area surface caused by cracking, heaving, settling, ponding, potholes, loose materials, erosion, rutting, etc that could cause tripping or falling.

SITE 15. Fencing and Gates
(2003 IPMC CROSS-REFERENCE: 302.7 ACCESSORY STRUCTURES)

DEFICIENCY: A fence or gate is rusted, deteriorated, or uprooted and may threaten security, health, or safety.

NOTE: Gates for swimming pool fences are covered in Other Items/Swimming Pool, Spa, or Whirlpool.

SITE 16. Condition
(2003 IPMC CROSS-REFERENCE: 302.1 SANITATION)

DEFICIENCY: Refuse, animal feces, broken glass/sharp edges, or holes/trip hazards are present.

SITE 17. Exposed Bolts
(2003 IPMC CROSS-REFERENCE: NONE)

DEFICIENCY: Playground equipment has exposed bolts.

SITE 18. Hanging or Choking Hazards
(2003 IPMC CROSS-REFERENCE: NONE)

DEFICIENCY: Playground equipment has hanging and/or choking hazards.

SITE 19. Open "S" Hooks
(2003 IPMC CROSS-REFERENCE: NONE)

DEFICIENCY: Swings or other playground equipment have open "S" hooks.

SITE 20. Pinch Hazards
(2003 IPMC CROSS-REFERENCE: NONE)

DEFICIENCY: Playground equipment has pinch hazards.

OTHER

SITE 21. Refuse Disposal
(2003 IPMC CROSS-REFERENCES: 307.2.1 RUBBISH STORAGE FACILITIES; 2003 IPMC CROSS-REFERENCE: 307.3.1 GARBAGE FACILITIES; 307.3.2 CONTAINERS)

Collection areas for common pickup of trash/garbage.

DEFICIENCY: Wall or roof for outdoor enclosed area is leaning or collapsed-OR-Concrete slab deteriorated-OR-Area is too small to store refuse until pickup-OR-Garbage cans are overflowing-OR-No exterior refuse disposal

NOTE: This does not include areas not designed as trash/refuse enclosures (such as curbside pick-up).

SITE 22. Retaining Walls
(2003 IPMC CROSS-REFERENCE: 304.6 EXTERIOR WALLS)

A wall built to support or prevent the advance of a mass of earth or water.

DEFICIENCY: A retaining wall structure is deteriorated, damaged, falling, or leaning.

SITE 23. Standing Water

(2003 IPMC CROSS-REFERENCE: NONE)

DEFICIENCY: Storm drainage areas (e.g., culverts, ditches) have standing water

SITE 24. Storm Drainage

(2003 IPMC CROSS-REFERENCES: 302.2 GRADING AND DRAINAGE; 507.1 GENERAL)

System used to collect and dispose of surface run-off water through the use of culverts, underground structures, or natural drainage features, e.g., swales, ditches, etc.

DEFICIENCY: Storm drainage system partially or completely blocked-OR-Runoffs into areas where runoffs are not intended.

SITE 25. Outdoor Water

(2003 IPMC CROSS-REFERENCE: NONE)

There is a pond, lake, stream, or drainage reservoir on site.

DEFICIENCY: Not necessarily a deficiency; assessed because condition could lead inspector to other issues.

SITE 26. Outdoor Water: Drainage Reservoir Fencing

(2003 IPMC CROSS-REFERENCE: NONE)

DEFICIENCY: Reservoir is not fully fenced or fence is damaged.

SITE 27. Septic Tank

(2003 IPMC CROSS-REFERENCE: NONE)

System used to treat wastewater on-site through use of holding tank/tile fields. Moist ground in the septic tank area is an imminent health hazard:
REPORT TO BUILDING MANAGEMENT/ OWNER IMMEDIATELY AND RECORD SPECIFICS IN THE COMMENTS SECTION.

DEFICIENCY: Moist ground in septic tank area.

NOTE: Do not identify a hazard if recent rain has made all of the ground moist.

SITE 28. Walkways/Steps/Hand Railing

(2003 IPMC CROSS-REFERENCES: 304.10 STAIRWAYS, DECKS, PORCHES AND BALCONIES; 304.12 HANDRAILS AND GUARDS; 306.1 GENERAL)

Passages for walking and the structures that allow for changes in vertical orientation. Deficiencies: broken/missing hand railing for four or more stairs, cracks/settlement/heaving, or spalling.

SITE 29. Large Trees

(2003 IPMC CROSS-REFERENCE: NONE)

DEFICIENCY: Large trees are hanging over and touching the unit.

BUILDING EXTERIOR (ITEMS 30–62)

Items to inspect in this category are
- Doors
- Fire escapes
- Foundations
- Lighting
- Roofs
- Walls
- Windows

EXTERIOR 30. Building Access for the Disabled

(2003 IPMC CROSS-REFERENCE: NONE)

DEFICIENCY: Building is not accessible for the disabled

NOTE: Not applicable in single-family units with no disabled residents.

DOORS

Means of access to the interior of a building or structure. Doors provide privacy, control passage, maintain security, and provide fire and weather resistance. Includes entry to maintenance areas, boiler and mechanical rooms, electrical vaults, storage areas, etc.

NOTE: This does not include unit doors, which are addressed in the Unit section.

EXTERIOR 31. Damaged Frames/Threshold/
Lintels/Trim
(2003 IPMC CROSS-REFERENCES: 304.15 DOORS; 304.13
WINDOW, SKYLIGHT AND DOOR FRAMES)

DEFICIENCY: A frame, header, jamb, threshold,
lintel, or trim is warped, split, cracked, or broken.

EXTERIOR 32. Damaged Hardware/Locks
(2003 IPMC CROSS-REFERENCES: 304.18 BUILDING SECURITY;
304.18.1 DOORS)

DEFICIENCIES: One or more exterior doors cannot
be locked: Door attachments that provide hinging,
hanging, opening, closing, or security are damaged
or missing. These include locks, panic hardware,
overhead door tracks, springs and pulleys, sliding
door tracks and hangers, and door closures.
This does not include storm doors.

NOTE: If a door is designed to have locks, the locks
should work. If a door is not designed to have locks,
do not record a deficiency for not having a lock.

EXTERIOR 33. Damaged Surface
(2003 IPMC CROSS-REFERENCE: 304.2 PROTECTIVE TREATMENT)

DEFICIENCY: Damage to a door surface that may
affect either the surface protection or the strength
of the door or may compromise building security.
This includes holes, peeling/cracking/no paint, broken
glass, and significant rust.

EXTERIOR 34. Screen/Storm Doors Damaged/Missing
(2003 IPMC CROSS-REFERENCE: 304.14 INSECT SCREENS)

DEFICIENCY: Surface damage on screen or storm
doors (includes screens, glass, frames, hardware, and
door surfaces)

EXTERIOR 35. Deteriorated/Missing Caulking/
Seals/Flashing
(2003 IPMC CROSS-REFERENCE: 304.2 PROTECTIVE TREATMENT)

DEFICIENCY: Sealant and stripping designed to
resist weather or caulking is missing or deteriorated.

NOTE: This applies only to entry doors that were
designed with seals. If a door shows evidence that
a seal was never part of its design, do not record a
deficiency.

EXTERIOR 36. Missing Doors
(in Exterior Doorways)
(2003 IPMC CROSS-REFERENCE: 304.15 DOORS)

DEFICIENCY: An exterior door is missing.

FIRE ESCAPES

EXTERIOR 37. Egress
(2003 IPMC CROSS-REFERENCES: 702.1 GENERAL; 702.2 AISLES;
702.3 LOCKED DOORS; 702.4 EMERGENCY ESCAPE OPENINGS)

All buildings must have acceptable fire exits. This
includes both stairway access doors and external exits.
These can include external fire escapes, fire towers,
operable windows on the lower floors with easy access
to the ground, or a back door opening onto a porch
with a stairway leading to the ground.

DEFICIENCY: Any part of the fire escape—including
ladders—is blocked, limiting or restricting people
from exiting-OR-In multifamily buildings, fire exits
are not properly marked-OR-A fire exit is cannot be
used or the exit is limited because a door or window
is nailed shut; a lock is broken; panic hardware is
chained; or debris, storage, or other conditions cause
the exit to be unusable.

NOTE: This includes fire escapes, fire towers, and
windows on the ground floor that would be used in
an emergency.

EXTERIOR 38. Components
(2003 IPMC CROSS-REFERENCE: 703.2 OPENING PROTECTIVES)

DEFICIENCY: Any of the components that affect the
function of the fire escape are missing.

EXTERIOR 39. Fire Escape
(2003 IPMC CROSS-REFERENCE: NONE)

DEFICIENCY: There is not at least one fire escape
for basements with bedrooms and finished living
spaces.

FOUNDATIONS

EXTERIOR 40. Foundation Type
(2003 IPMC CROSS-REFERENCE: NONE)

Foundations can be slabs, crawl spaces, basements, or cellars.

DEFICIENCY: Not necessarily a deficiency; assessed because type of foundation could lead inspector to other issues.

EXTERIOR 41. Cracks/Gaps
(2003 IPMC CROSS-REFERENCE: 304.5 FOUNDATION WALLS)

Lowest level structural wall or floor responsible for transferring the building's load to the appropriate footings and soil. Materials may include concrete, stone, masonry, and wood. This inspectable item can have the following deficiencies: cracks/gaps, spalling/exposed rebar, or bulging.

NOTE: Cracks that show evidence of water penetration should be evaluated here. If there is any doubt about the severity of the problem, request an inspection by a structural engineer. A bulged foundation (to the interior) often signals a serious structural problem.

EXTERIOR 42. Spalling/Exposed Rebar
(2003 IPMC CROSS-REFERENCE: 304.5 FOUNDATION WALLS)

DEFICIENCY: A concrete or masonry wall is flaking, chipping, or crumbling, possibly exposing underlying reinforcing material (rebar).

NOTE: If there is any doubt about the severity of the problem, request an inspection by a structural engineer.

LIGHTING

EXTERIOR 43. Fixtures/Bulbs
(2003 IPMC CROSS-REFERENCE: NONE)

System to provide illumination of building exteriors and surrounding grounds. Includes fixtures, lamps, stanchions, poles, supports, and electrical supply that are associated with the building itself. This covers all or part of the lighting associated with the building, including lighting attached to the building used to light the site. If a lighting fixture present is not directly attached to a specific building, assign it to the nearest building. If there are areas in need of exterior lighting or areas with no exterior lighting, check the box for no exterior lighting.

NOTE: IF THE CONDITION CONSTITUTES AN OBVIOUS SAFETY HAZARD: REPORT TO BUILDING MANAGEMENT/OWNER IMMEDIATELY AND RECORD SPECIFICS IN THE COMMENTS SECTION. This includes broken fixtures and bulbs that could fall on pedestrians or lead to electrocution.

ROOFS

The roof system consists of the structural deck, weathering surface, flashing, parapet, and drainage system. Roofs may be flat or pitched. This inspectable item can have the following deficiencies: damaged/clogged drains, damaged soffits/fascia, damaged vents, damaged/torn membrane/missing ballast, missing/damaged components from downspout/gutter, missing/damaged shingles, or ponding (roofs)

EXTERIOR 44. Damaged/Clogged Drains
(2003 IPMC CROSS-REFERENCE: 304.7 ROOFS AND DRAINAGE)

DEFICIENCY: The drainage system does not effectively remove water. Generally, this deficiency applies to flat roofs.

If there has been measurable precipitation (1/10 inch or more) during the previous 48 hours, consider its impact on the extent of any ponding. Determine that ponding has occurred only when there is clear evidence—e.g., staining—of a persistent or longstanding problem. Keep in mind that some flat roofs are designed to allow ponding.

NOTE: If there is any doubt about the severity of the condition, an inspection by a roofing specialist is recommended.

EXTERIOR 45. Chimney Clearance
(2003 IPMC CROSS-REFERENCE: NONE)

DEFICIENCY: Chimney height is less than 3 feet above the highest point where the chimney penetrates the roofline.

EXTERIOR 46. Damaged Soffits/Fascia/Flashing
(2003 IPMC CROSS-REFERENCES: 304.7 ROOFS AND
DRAINAGE; 304.8 DECORATIVE FEATURES)

DEFICIENCY: Damage to soffit, fascia, soffit vents, or associated components that may provide opportunity for water penetration or other damage from natural elements.

NOTE: If there is any doubt about the severity of the condition, an inspection by a roofing specialist is recommended.

EXTERIOR 47. Vents
(2003 IPMC CROSS-REFERENCE: 304.7 ROOFS AND DRAINAGE)

DEFICIENCY: Damaged vents on or extending through the roof surface or damaged or missing vent components. Vents include ridge vents, gable vents, plumbing vents, gas vents, and other vents as well as their flashings.

EXTERIOR 48. Gutters/Downspouts
(2003 IPMC CROSS-REFERENCE: 304.7 ROOFS AND DRAINAGE)

DEFICIENCY: Components of the drainage system—including gutters, leaders, downspouts, splash-blocks, and drain openings—are missing or damaged. Check for proper grading away from building.

NOTES: Jurisdictions may wish to consider expressing roof damage for larger roof surfaces as a percentage.

EXTERIOR 49. Gutters/Downspout Discharge
(2003 IPMC CROSS-REFERENCE: NONE)

DEFICIENCY: The gutter/downspout grading and/or discharge point is such that water will pool toward the building, instead of away from the building, increasing the likelihood of basement and foundation leaks.

EXTERIOR 50. Shingles or Tiles or Other Roofing Material
(2003 IPMC CROSS-REFERENCE: 304.7 ROOFS AND DRAINAGE)

DEFICIENCY: Shingles, tiles, or other roofing materials are missing or damaged, including cracking, warping, cupping, and other deterioration.

NOTE: If there is any doubt about the severity of the condition, an inspection by a roofing specialist is recommended. Do not climb on sloped roof: look at the roof from the street.

WALLS

The exterior enclosure of the building or structure. Materials for construction include concrete, masonry block, brick, stone, wood, and glass block. Surface finish materials include metal, wood, vinyl, and stucco.

NOTE: This does not include foundation walls. This inspectable item can have the following deficiencies: cracks/gaps, damaged chimneys, missing pieces/holes/spalling, missing/damaged caulking/mortar, or stained/peeling/needs paint.

EXTERIOR 51. Primary Exterior Wall Surfaces
(2003 IPMC CROSS-REFERENCE: NONE)
Surfaces can be built of brick, stucco, wood, stone, cement/concrete block, asbestos, vinyl, or other materials.

DEFICIENCY: Not necessarily a deficiency; assessed because type of surface could lead inspector to other issues.

EXTERIOR 52. Secondary Exterior Wall Surfaces
(2003 IPMC CROSS-REFERENCE: NONE)
Surfaces can be built of brick, stucco, wood, stone, cement/concrete block, asbestos, vinyl, or other materials.

DEFICIENCY: Not necessarily a deficiency; assessed because type of surface could lead inspector to other issues.

EXTERIOR 53. Wall Cracks and Gaps
(2003 IPMC CROSS-REFERENCES: 304.1 GENERAL; 304.2 PROTECTIVE TREATMENT)

DEFICIENCY: There is a split, separation, or gap in the exterior walls.

NOTE: If there is any doubt about the severity of the condition, request an inspection by a structural engineer.

EXTERIOR 54. Damaged Chimney
(2003 IPMC CROSS-REFERENCE: 304.11 CHIMNEYS AND TOWERS)

DEFICIENCY: The chimney, including the part that extends above the roof line, has separated from the wall or has cracks, spalling, missing pieces, or broken sections.

EXTERIOR 55. Wall Surface Deterioration
(2003 IPMC CROSS-REFERENCES: 304.1 GENERAL;
304.2 PROTECTIVE TREATMENT)

DEFICIENCY: There is deterioration of the exterior wall surface, including missing pieces, holes, or spalling. This may also be attributed to rotting materials -OR-a concrete, stucco, or masonry wall that is flaking, chipping, or crumbling.

NOTE: If there is any doubt about the severity of the condition, request an inspection by a structural engineer.

EXTERIOR 56. Masonry Caulking and/or Mortar
(2003 IPMC CROSS-REFERENCES: 304.1 GENERAL;
304.2 PROTECTIVE TREATMENT)

DEFICIENCY: Caulking designed to resist weather or mortar is missing or deteriorated.

NOTE: This does not include caulking relative to doors and windows; they are covered in other areas. Address all other caulking here.

EXTERIOR 57. Wall, Soffit, Fascia Paint/Water Damage
(2003 IPMC CROSS-REFERENCES: 304.1 GENERAL;
304.2 PROTECTIVE TREATMENT)

DEFICIENCY: Paint is cracking, flaking, or otherwise deteriorated or any exterior building surface, such as (but not limited to) walls, soffits, and fascia. Water damage or related problems have stained the paint.

NOTE: This does not include walls that are not intended to have paint, such as most brick walls. An areas of deteriorated exterior paint larger than 20 square feet that contains 1 mg/cm² of lead or more is defined in regulations as a significant (non-de minimis) lead-based paint hazard in most pre-1978 housing.

WINDOWS

Window systems provide light, security, and exclusion of exterior noise, dust, heat, and cold. Frame materials include wood, aluminum, and vinyl. This inspectable item can have the following deficiencies: broken/missing/cracked panes, damaged/missing screens, damaged sills/frames/lintels/trim, missing/deteriorated caulking/seals/glazing compound, peeling/needs paint, or security bars prevent egress.

NOTE: This does not include windows that have defects noted from inspection inside the unit.

EXTERIOR 58. Window Panes
(2003 IPMC CROSS-REFERENCE: 304.13 WINDOW, SKYLIGHT
AND DOOR FRAMES)

DEFICIENCY: A glass pane is broken, missing, or cracked.

EXTERIOR 59. Screens
(2003 IPMC CROSS-REFERENCE: 304.14 INSECT SCREENS)

DEFICIENCY: Screens are punctured, torn, otherwise damaged, or missing.

EXTERIOR 60. Sills/Frames/Lintels/Trim
(2003 IPMC CROSS-REFERENCE: 304.13 WINDOW, SKYLIGHT
AND DOOR FRAMES)

DEFICIENCY: Exterior window sills, frames, sash lintels, or trim are damaged by decay, rust, rot, corrosion, or other deterioration.

NOTE: Damage does not include scratches and cosmetic deficiencies.

EXTERIOR 61. Caulking/Seals/Glazing Compound
(2003 IPMC CROSS-REFERENCE: 304.13.1 GLAZING)

DEFICIENCY: The caulking or glazing compound that resists weather is missing or deteriorated.

NOTE: This also includes insulated windows that have failed. Caulk and seals are considered to be deteriorated when two or more seals for any window have lost their elasticity. (If the seals crumble and flake when touched, they have lost their elasticity.)

EXTERIOR 62. Window Assembly or Trim Paint
(2003 IPMC CROSS-REFERENCE: 304.2 PROTECTIVE
TREATMENT)

DEFICIENCY: Paint covering the window assembly or trim is cracking, flaking, or otherwise failing -OR- The window assembly or trim is not painted or is exposed to the elements.

NOTE: This does not include windows that are not intended to be painted. Paint that is lead based and more than 10% deteriorated is defined in regulations as a significant (non-de minimis) lead-based paint hazard.

BUILDING SYSTEMS (ITEMS 63–81)
Items to inspect in this category (multihome sites only) include

- Electrical Systems
- Fire Protection
- HVAC

BUILDING SYSTEMS 63. Central Water Supply or Sewage System
(2003 IPMC CROSS-REFERENCES: 504.1 GENERAL;
603.1 MECHANICAL APPLIANCES)

The portion of the building system that provides potable water conditioning, heating, and distribution, taking its source from outside the building and terminating in domestic plumbing fixtures and drains. The system typically consists of water conditioners (filters and softeners), water heaters, transfer and circulating pumps, strainers, and connecting piping, fittings, valves, and supports and drains. **IF LEAKING WATER IS A SAFETY CONCERN (I.E., IS LEAKING ON OR NEAR ELECTRICAL EQUIPMENT), REPORT IT TO BUILDING MANAGEMENT/OWNER IMMEDIATELY AND RECORD SPECIFICS IN THE COMMENTS SECTION.**

NOTE: This does not include portion of water supply that connects to the heating and cooling system or the delivery points of the system such as sinks and faucets in units or common areas.
This inspectable item can have the following deficiencies: leaking central water supply and sewage systems, misaligned/damaged ventilation systems, missing pressure relief valve, or rust/corrosion on heater chimney.

DEFICIENCY: Water leaking from any water system component, including valve flanges, stems, bodies, hose bibs, or any domestic water tank or its pipe or pipe connections.

NOTE: This includes both hot and cold water systems but does not include fixtures. Fixtures are covered in the Unit section. Some pumps and valves are designed to leak, particularly in fire pumps, water pressure pumps, and large circulating pumps, and should be considered accordingly.

BUILDING SYSTEMS 64. Outside Water Spigots
(2003 IPMC CROSS-REFERENCE: NONE)

DEFICIENCY: Outside water spigots should be protected by hose bibb vacuum breakers; however, this is not necessarily a code requirement in all areas.

BUILDING SYSTEMS 65. Chimney Exhaust Ventilation for Fuel-Fired Equipment
(2003 IPMC CROSS-REFERENCE: 603.2 REMOVAL OF
COMBUSTION PRODUCTS)

DEFICIENCY: The ventilation system on a gas-fired or oil-fired water heater is misaligned-OR-There is no pressure relief valve.

BUILDING SYSTEMS 66. Makeup Air
(2003 IPMC CROSS-REFERENCE: NONE)

DEFICIENCY: Makeup air is not provided to the fireplace, gas water heater, or fuel-burning fixtures.

ELECTRICAL SYSTEMS (BUILDING)
BUILDING SYSTEMS 67. Breakers/Fuses
(2003 IPMC CROSS-REFERENCE: 605.1 INSTALLATION)
Portion of the building system that safely provides electrical power throughout the building, including equipment that provides control, protection, metering, and service.

NOTE: This does not include transformers or metering that belongs to the providing utility, equipment that is part of any emergency power generating system, or terminal equipment such as receptacles, switches, or panelboards located in the units or common areas (which are inspected in the Unit or Common Area sections).

This inspectable item can have the following deficiencies: blocked access/improper storage, burnt or melted or missing breakers or improper fusing, evidence of leaks/corrosion, frayed wiring, missing breakers/fuses, or missing covers.

DEFICIENCY: Breakers have carbon on the plastic body or the plastic body is melted or scarred.

NOTE: Do not attempt to disassemble any electrical component or touch any circuit.

BUILDING SYSTEMS 68. Water Leaks or Corrosion On or Near Electrical Systems
(2003 IPMC CROSS-REFERENCE: 605.1 INSTALLATION)

DEFICIENCY: There are liquid stains, rust marks, or other signs of corrosion on electrical enclosures or hardware.

NOTE: Do not consider surface rust a deficiency if it does not affect the condition of the electrical enclosure.

BUILDING SYSTEMS 69. Wiring
(2003 IPMC CROSS-REFERENCE: 605.1 INSTALLATION)

DEFICIENCY: There are nicks, abrasions, or fraying of the insulation exposing wires that conduct current.

NOTE: Do not consider this a deficiency for wires that are not intended to be insulated, such as grounding wires.

BUILDING SYSTEMS 70. Extension Cord Use
(2003 IPMC CROSS-REFERENCE: NONE)

DEFICIENCY: Extension cords are not used properly (are draped over doorways or under carpets) or are overloaded with multiple appliances.

BUILDING SYSTEMS 71. Extension Cord Condition
(2003 IPMC CROSS-REFERENCE: NONE)

DEFICIENCY: Extension cords are cracked or frayed.

BUILDING SYSTEMS 72. Electrical covers
(2003 IPMC CROSS-REFERENCE: 605.1 INSTALLATION)

DEFICIENCY: The cover is missing from any electrical device box, panel box, switch gear box, or control panel with exposed electrical connections-OR-In a panel board, main panel board, or other electrical box containing circuit breakers, an open circuit breaker position is not appropriately blanked off.

NOTE: If the accompanying authority identifies abandoned wiring, capped wires do not pose a risk; therefore, do not record this as a deficiency.

FIRE PROTECTION (BUILDING)
Building systems designed to minimize the effects of a fire. These systems include fire walls and doors, portable fire extinguishers, and permanent sprinkler systems.

NOTE: This does not include fire detection, alarm, and control devices.

This inspectable item can have the following deficiencies: missing or disabled sprinkler head or missing/damaged/expired extinguishers.

BUILDING SYSTEMS 73. Fire Sprinklers
(2003 IPMC CROSS-REFERENCE: 704.1 GENERAL)

DEFICIENCY: A sprinkler head—or its components—connected to the central fire protection system is missing, visibly disabled, painted over, blocked, capped, or otherwise disabled. **REPORT TO BUILDING MANAGEMENT/OWNER IMMEDIATELY AND RECORD SPECIFICS IN THE COMMENTS SECTION.**

NOTE: Components include test plugs, drains, and test fittings.

BUILDING SYSTEMS 74. Missing, Damaged, Expired or Wrong Kind of Fire Extinguishers/Fire Hoses
(2003 IPMC CROSS-REFERENCE: 704.1 GENERAL)

DEFICIENCY: A portable fire extinguisher is not where it should be or is damaged-OR-Fire extinguisher certification is expired-OR-Fire extinguisher is the wrong kind. Fire extinguishers for homes should use dry chemicals and be effective on Class A, B, and C fires. **IF THERE ARE NO FIRE EXTIN-GUISHERS, REPORT TO BUILDING MANAGE-MENT/OWNER IMMEDIATELY AND RECORD SPECIFICS IN THE COMMENTS SECTION.**

NOTE: This includes missing/damaged fire hoses where there are fire cabinets. For buildings with multiple fire-control systems (standpipes, sprinklers, etc.), less than 1% of the extinguishers for a given building may be missing, damaged, and/or expired. In those cases, do not record as a deficiency. If the inspection tag is missing during the inspection, the accompanying authority may produce proof that the fire extinguisher certification is current. If such proof is provided, do not record a deficiency for a missing tag.

BUILDING SYSTEMS 75. Emergency Exit/Egress Routes

DEFICIENCY: Emergency exit routes are not clear of furniture, toys, or clutter.

HVAC (BUILDING)

Portion of the building system that provides ability to heat or cool the air within the building. Includes equipment such as boilers, burners, furnaces, fuel supply, hot water and steam distribution, and associated piping, filters, and equipment. Also includes air handling equipment and associated ventilation ducting.

This inspectable items can have the following deficiencies: boiler/pump leaks, fuel supply leaks, misaligned chimney/ventilation systems, or general rust/corrosion.

BUILDING SYSTEMS 76. Boiler/Pump
(2003 IPMC CROSS-REFERENCE: 603.1 MECHANICAL APPLIANCES)

DEFICIENCY: Water or steam is escaping from unit casing or system piping or boiler

NOTE: Also do not include steam escaping from pressure relief valves.

BUILDING SYSTEMS 77. Fuel Supply
(2003 IPMC CROSS-REFERENCE: NONE)

DEFICIENCY: There is evidence that fuel is escaping from a fuel storage tank or fuel line. **REPORT LEAKS TO BUILDING MANAGEMENT/OWNER IMMEDIATELY AND RECORD SPECIFICS IN THE COMMENTS SECTION. THE ODOR OF NATURAL GAS OR PROPANE IS AN IMMINENT HEALTH HAZARD; THE STRUCTURE SHOULD BE EVACUATED.**

BUILDING SYSTEMS 78. Chimney Exhaust
(2003 IPMC CROSS-REFERENCE: 603.2 REMOVAL OF COMBUSTION PRODUCTS)

DEFICIENCY: The exhaust system on a gas-fired or oil-fired unit is misaligned, blocked, rusted, disconnected, or corroded-OR-There is reverse air flow in chimney. If reverse air flow is observed, report to building management/owner immediately and record specifics in the comments section.

BUILDING SYSTEMS 79. Chimney Spark Arrestor and Rain Cap
(2003 IPMC CROSS-REFERENCE: NONE)

DEFICIENCY: A chimney spark arrestor and rain cap are not installed.

BUILDING SYSTEMS 80. HVAC Condensate and Sewage Corrosion
(2003 IPMC CROSS-REFERENCES: 603.1 MECHANICAL APPLIANCES; 506.2 MAINTENANCE)

DEFICIENCY: HVAC equipment, condensate systems, associated piping and ducting, and sewage system shows evidence of flaking, discoloration, pitting, corrosion, or crevices. The sewage system includes that portion of the building system that provides for the disposal of waste products with discharge to the local sewage system. This can include sources such as domestic plumbing fixtures; floor drains, traps; and other area drains; collection sumps; sewage ejectors and pumps; and collection piping, fittings, valves, and supports.

BUILDING SYSTEMS 81. HVAC Air Supply

(2003 IPMC CROSS-REFERENCE: NONE)

DEFICIENCY: All supply air for the HVAC system is drawn from the basement, with no functioning return air systems from living areas. Determine whether there is a source of fresh air delivered to the HVAC system (this does not include building leakage and/or open windows or doors).

COMMON AREAS (ITEMS 82–102)

Items to inspect in this section (multihome sites only) include

- Walkways/steps
- Ceiling
- Floor

ELEVATORS

COMMON AREAS 82. Elevators

(2003 IPMC CROSS-REFERENCE: NONE)

DEFICIENCY: Elevators and elevator equipment do not work properly.

SIGNAGE

COMMON AREAS 83. Exit Signage

(2003 IPMC CROSS-REFERENCE: NONE)

DEFICIENCY: Exit signs should be visible and not broken.

SMOKING AREAS

COMMON AREAS 84. Designated Smoking Area

(2003 IPMC CROSS-REFERENCE: NONE)

DEFICIENCY: The area is littered with cigarette butts or food debris.

INTERIOR TRASH

COMMON AREAS 85. Trash Collection Areas

(2003 IPMC CROSS-REFERENCE: 307.1 ACCUMULATION OF RUBBISH OR GARBAGE)

Interior collection areas for trash/garbage common pick-up or conveyance.

DEFICIENCIES: Trash on common area floor, containers missing covers or not sealed, or trash chutes damaged or missing components.

OUTLETS, SWITCHES, COVER PLATES

COMMON AREAS 86. Electrical Outlets

(2003 IPMC CROSS-REFERENCE: 605.2 RECEPTACLES)
The receptacle connected to a power supply or method to control the flow of electricity. This includes two- and three-prong outlets, ground fault circuit interrupters, pull cords, two- and three-pole switches, and dimmer switches.

This inspectable item can have the following deficiencies: missing/broken wiring or exposed wiring.

SMOKE AND CARBON MONOXIDE DETECTORS

COMMON AREAS 87. Smoke Detectors

(2003 IPMC CROSS-REFERENCE: 704.2 SMOKE ALARMS)

Sensor to detect the presence of smoke and activate an alarm. May be battery operated or hard-wired to electrical system.

This inspectable item can have the following deficiency: missing/inoperable.

COMMON AREAS 88. Carbon Monoxide Detectors

(2003 IPMC CROSS-REFERENCE: NONE)
Sensor to detect the presence of carbon monoxide and activate an alarm. May be battery operated or hard-wired to electrical system.

This inspectable item can have the following deficiency: missing/inoperable.

WALKWAYS/STEPS

COMMON AREAS 89. Walkways/Steps

(2003 IPMC CROSS-REFERENCES: 305.4 STAIRS AND WALKING SURFACES; 305.5 HANDRAILS AND GUARDS; 306.1 GENERAL)

DEFICIENCY: Walkways or steps damaged or broken or missing handrailing

CEILING

COMMON AREAS 90. Ceiling Buckling
(2003 IPMC CROSS-REFERENCE: 305.3 INTERIOR SURFACES)

The visible overhead structure lining the inside of a room or area.

This inspectable item can have the following deficiencies: bulging/buckling, holes/missing tiles/panels/cracks, peeling/needs paint, or water stains/water damage/mold/mildew.

DEFICIENCY: A ceiling is bowed, deflected, sagging, or is no longer aligned horizontally.

NOTE: If there is any doubt about the severity of the condition, request an inspection by a structural engineer.

COMMON AREAS 91. Ceiling Holes
(2003 IPMC CROSS-REFERENCE: 305.3 INTERIOR SURFACES)

DEFICIENCY: The ceiling surface has punctures that may or may not penetrate completely-OR-Panels or tiles are missing or damaged.

COMMON AREAS 92. Peeling/Needs Paint
(2003 IPMC CROSS-REFERENCE: 305.3 INTERIOR SURFACES)

DEFICIENCY: Paint is peeling, cracking, flaking, or otherwise deteriorated on ceilings in common areas. Note: Paint that is lead-based and larger than 2 square feet in area is defined in regulations as a significant (non-de minimis) lead-based paint hazard.

COMMON AREAS 93. Water Stains/Water Damage
(2003 IPMC CROSS-REFERENCE: 305.3 INTERIOR SURFACES)

DEFICIENCY: There is evidence of water infiltration or leaks such as water stains (but not mold) that may have been caused by saturation or surface failure. Water or moisture may or may not be visible.

COMMON AREAS 94. Mold
(2003 IPMC CROSS-REFERENCE: 305.3 INTERIOR SURFACES)

DEFICIENCY: There is evidence of mold or mildew (such as a darkening of the surface) that may have been caused by saturation, surface failure, leaks, condensation, etc.-OR-There is a moldy or musty odor.

COMMON AREAS 95. Mold Source
(2003 IPMC CROSS-REFERENCE: NONE)

DEFICIENCY: There is a leaking roof or appliance or water pipe in wall or ceiling.

FLOORS

Floors are defined as the visible horizontal surface system within a room or area underfoot; the horizontal division between two stories of a structure.

This inspectable item can have the following deficiencies: bulging/buckling, floor covering damaged, missing flooring/tiles, peeling/needs paint, rot/deteriorated subfloor, or water stains/water damage/mold/mildew.

COMMON AREAS 96. Floor Buckling
(2003 IPMC CROSS-REFERENCES: 305.3 INTERIOR SURFACES; 305.2 STRUCTURAL MEMBERS)

DEFICIENCY: The floor is bowed, deflected, sagging, or is no longer aligned horizontally.

COMMON AREAS 97. Floor Covering
(2003 IPMC CROSS-REFERENCE: 305.3 INTERIOR SURFACES)

DEFICIENCY: There is damage to carpet, carpet tiles, wood, sheet vinyl, or other floor covering.

COMMON AREAS 98. Flooring/Tiles
(2003 IPMC CROSS-REFERENCE: 305.3 INTERIOR SURFACES)

DEFICIENCY: Flooring (terrazo, hardwood, ceramic tile, or other flooring material) is missing or damaged.

NOTE: If there is just one concern that safety is compromised, classify the floor system as >50% missing.

COMMON AREAS 99. Peeling/Deteriorated Paint
(2003 IPMC CROSS-REFERENCE: 305.3 INTERIOR SURFACES)

DEFICIENCY: On painted floors, paint is peeling, cracking, flaking, or otherwise deteriorated or separating from the substrate.

NOTE: Paint that is lead-based and larger than 2 square feet in area is defined in regulations as a significant lead-based paint hazard.

COMMON AREAS 100. Subfloor
(2003 IPMC CROSS-REFERENCE: 305.2 STRUCTURAL MEMBERS)

DEFICIENCY: The subfloor has decayed or is decaying.

COMMON AREAS 101. Water Stains/Water Damage
(2003 IPMC CROSS-REFERENCE: 305.3 INTERIOR SURFACES)

DEFICIENCY: There is evidence of water infiltration or stains that may have been caused by saturation or surface failure or leaks. Record mold on floor in Common Areas 102: Mold.

COMMON AREAS 102. Mold
(2003 IPMC CROSS-REFERENCE: 305.3 INTERIOR SURFACES)

DEFICIENCY: There is evidence of mold or mildew (such as a darkening of the surface) that may have been caused by saturation, surface failure, leaks, or condensation.

HOUSING UNIT (ITEMS 103–196)
Items to inspect in the Housing Unit are as follows:
- Bathroom
- Ceiling, floors, and walls
- Doors
- Electrical
- Water heater
- HVAC system
- Kitchen
- Laundry area
- Lighting
- Patio/porch/deck/balcony
- Smoke and carbon monoxide detectors
- Stairs
- Windows

BATHROOM
A room equipped with a water closet or toilet, tub and/or shower, sink, cabinet(s), and/or closet.

This inspectable item can have the following deficiencies: damaged or missing bathroom cabinets or lavatory sink; clogged drains; leaking faucet or pipes; damaged or missing shower or tub; inoperable ventilation or exhaust systems; damaged, clogged, or missing water closet or toilet; or permanent carpet on bathroom floor.

HOUSING UNIT 103. Bathroom Cabinets
(2003 IPMC CROSS-REFERENCE: 403.2 BATHROOMS AND TOILET ROOMS)

DEFICIENCY: There are damaged or missing cabinets, vanity tops, drawers, shelves, doors, medicine cabinets, or vanities.

HOUSING UNIT 104. Lavatory Sink
(2003 IPMC CROSS-REFERENCE: 504.1 GENERAL)

DEFICIENCY: A basin (sink) is missing or shows signs of deterioration or distress.

NOTE: If the stopper is near the shower/tub area, do not record it as a deficiency.

HOUSING UNIT 105. Plumbing Drain
(2003 IPMC CROSS-REFERENCE: 504.1 GENERAL)

DEFICIENCY: Water does not drain adequately in the shower, tub, or basin (sink).

HOUSING UNIT 106. Plumbing Faucets/Fixtures
(2003 IPMC CROSS-REFERENCE: 504.1 GENERAL)

DEFICIENCY: A basin, shower, water closet, tub faucet, or associated pipes are leaking water.

HOUSING UNIT 107. Water Temperature
(2003 IPMC CROSS-REFERENCE: NONE)

DEFICIENCY: Hot and cold water are not both present-OR-Hot water temperature is >120°F.

HOUSING UNIT 108. Water Pressure

(2003 IPMC CROSS-REFERENCE: NONE)

DEFICIENCY: All bathroom plumbing fixtures do not have adequate water pressure.

HOUSING UNIT 109. Shower/Tub Surface

(2003 IPMC CROSS-REFERENCE: 505.1 GENERAL)

DEFICIENCY: The shower, tub, or components are damaged or missing. This includes associated hardware such as shower doors, functioning shower enclosure, or shower curtain.

NOTE: If there is a stopper near the shower/tub area, do not record it as a deficiency.

HOUSING UNIT 110. Shower/Tub Grab Bars

(2003 IPMC CROSS-REFERENCE: NONE)

DEFICIENCY: Grab bars are not properly installed inside and outside of shower/tub. This item applies to households with elderly residents or a resident with a physical handicap.

HOUSING UNIT 111. Bathroom Exhaust

(2003 IPMC CROSS-REFERENCE: 403.2 BATHROOMS AND TOILET ROOMS)

DEFICIENCY: Bathroom exhaust fan is not working or not present.

NOTE: If a resident has blocked an exhaust fan but it can function properly, do not record this as a deficiency. If a resident has disconnected a fan, consider it functional if it can be immediately reconnected for inspection. Record the absence of a fan even it there is a window in the bathroom.

HOUSING UNIT 112. Toilet

(2003 IPMC CROSS-REFERENCE: 504.1 GENERAL)

DEFICIENCY: A water closet/toilet is damaged or missing. **IF A HAZARDOUS CONDITION IS OBSERVED, REPORT TO BUILDING MANAGEMENT/OWNER IMMEDIATELY AND RECORD SPECIFICS IN THE COMMENTS SECTION.**

HOUSING UNIT 113. Toilet Grab Bars

(2003 IPMC CROSS-REFERENCE: NONE)

DEFICIENCY: Toilet grab bars are not properly installed next to toilet. This item applies to households with elderly residents or a resident with a physical handicap.

HOUSING UNIT 114. Shower/Bath/Toilet Caulking and/or Seals

(2003 IPMC CROSS-REFERENCE: NONE)

DEFICIENCY: Caulking and/or seals on shower, bath, or toilet are deteriorated.

HOUSING UNIT 115. Bathroom Call-for-Aid

(2003 IPMC CROSS-REFERENCE: NONE)

Systems to summon help. These systems can be visual, audible, or both. They may be activated manually or automatically when preprogrammed conditions are met. This inspectable item can have the following deficiency: inoperable or missing. This item applies to households with elderly residents or a resident with a physical handicap.

DEFICIENCY: The system does not function as it should or is absent

HOUSING UNIT 116. Permanent Carpet on Bathroom Floor

(2003 IPMC CROSS-REFERENCE: NONE)

DEFICIENCY: A permanent carpet, such as wall-to-wall carpet, is present in the bathroom, limiting drying and cleaning. This does not include bath mats and throw rugs that can be removed for cleaning and drying.

CEILING, FLOORS, AND WALLS

The inside envelope inside the housing unit, including the visible overhead structure lining the inside of a room or area (ceiling), the walls, and the floors and associated trim (e.g., baseboards, cove molding, chair rail, base molding, or other decorative trim). This inspectable item can have the following deficiencies: bulging/buckling, holes/missing tiles/panels/cracks, peeling/needs paint, or water stains/water damage/mold/mildew.

HOUSING UNIT 117. Bulging/Buckling
(2003 IPMC CROSS-REFERENCE: 305.3 INTERIOR SURFACES)

DEFICIENCY: The ceiling, walls, or floors are bowed, deflected, sagging, or are no longer aligned horizontally or vertically.

NOTE: If there is any doubt about the severity of the condition, request an inspection by a structural engineer.

HOUSING UNIT 118. Holes
(2003 IPMC CROSS-REFERENCE: 305.3 INTERIOR SURFACES)

DEFICIENCY: The ceiling, walls, or floor surfaces have punctures that may or may not penetrate completely-OR-Panels or tiles are missing or damaged. This does not include small holes created by hanging pictures, etc.

HOUSING UNIT 119. Peeling/Needs Paint
(2003 IPMC CROSS-REFERENCE: 305.3 INTERIOR SURFACES)

DEFICIENCY: Paint is peeling, cracking, flaking, or otherwise deteriorated.

NOTE: Paint that is lead-based and larger than 2 square feet in area in any one room is defined in regulations as a significant (non-deminimis) lead-based paint hazard.

HOUSING UNIT 120. Water Stains/Water Damage
(2003 IPMC CROSS-REFERENCE: 305.3 INTERIOR SURFACES)

DEFICIENCY: There is evidence of water infiltration, mold, or mildew that may have been caused by saturation or surface failure. Record mold or mildew in Housing Unit 122: Mold.

HOUSING UNIT 121. Condensation on Windows
(2003 IPMC CROSS-REFERENCE: NONE)

There is condensation on windows, doors, or walls.

HOUSING UNIT 122. Mold
(2003 IPMC CROSS-REFERENCE: 305.3 INTERIOR SURFACES)

DEFICIENCY: There is evidence of mold or mildew (such as a darkening of the surface) that may have been caused by saturation, surface failure, leaks, condensation, etc.-OR-There is a musty odor.

HOUSING UNIT 123. Mold Source
(2003 IPMC CROSS-REFERENCE: NONE)

There is a leaking roof or appliance or water pipe in wall or ceiling.

DOORS

Means of access to the interior of a unit, room within the unit, or closet. Doors provide privacy and security, control passage, provide fire and weather resistance. This inspectable item can have the following deficiencies: damaged surface (holes/paint/rusting/glass), damaged frames/threshold/lintels/trim, damaged hardware/locks, damaged/missing screen/storm/security door, deteriorated/missing seals (entry only), or missing door.

HOUSING UNIT 124. Door Surface
(2003 IPMC CROSS-REFERENCES: 305.6 INTERIOR DOORS; 305.3 INTERIOR SURFACES)

DEFICIENCY: There is damage to the door surface that may affect either the surface protection or the strength of the door-OR-that may compromise building security. This includes holes, peeling/cracking/no paint, broken glass, and significant rust.

HOUSING UNIT 125. Frame/Threshold/Lintel/Trim
(2003 IPMC CROSS-REFERENCE: 305.6 INTERIOR DOORS)

DEFICIENCY: There is a frame, header, jamb, threshold, lintel, or trim that is warped, split, cracked, or broken-OR-There is damage to a door's hardware (locks, hinges, etc.) If a door is designed to have a lock, the lock should work. If a door is designed without locks, do not record it as a deficiency. If a lock has been removed from an interior door, do not record it as a deficiency. Do not attempt to open a closed door within a housing unit without the permission of the resident and/or accompanying authority.

HOUSING UNIT 126. Seals (Entry Only)
(2003 IPMC CROSS-REFERENCE: 305.6 INTERIOR DOORS)

DEFICIENCY: The seals and stripping around the entry door(s) to resist weather and fire are damaged or missing.

NOTE: This defect applies only to entry doors that were designed with seals. If a door shows evidence that a seal was never part of its design, do not record it as a deficiency.

HOUSING UNIT 127. Door Missing
(2003 IPMC CROSS-REFERENCE: 305.6 INTERIOR DOORS)

DEFICIENCY: A door is missing.

NOTE: If a bathroom or entry door is missing, record it as a deficiency. If a bedroom door has been removed to improve access for an elderly or handicapped resident, do not record it as a deficiency.

HOUSING UNIT 128. Deadbolt Locks
(2003 IPMC CROSS-REFERENCE: NONE)

DEFICIENCY: Deadbolt locks cannot be unlocked from the inside without a key.

HOUSING UNIT 129. Door Lock Operation
(2003 IPMC CROSS-REFERENCE: NONE)

DEFICIENCY: Door locks cannot be operated by a child in an emergency.

ELECTRICAL
Portion of the unit that safely provides electrical power throughout the building. Includes equipment that provides control, protection, metering, and service. This inspectable item can have the following deficiencies: blocked access to electric panel, burnt breakers, evidence of leaks or corrosion, frayed wiring, inoperable ground fault circuit interruptor, missing breakers/fuses, or missing covers.

HOUSING UNIT 130. Electrical Panel Access
(2003 IPMC CROSS-REFERENCE: 605.1 INSTALLATION)

DEFICIENCY: A fixed obstruction or item of sufficient size and weight that can delay or prevent access to any panel board switch in an emergency.

NOTE: If there is an easy-to-remove item, like a picture, do not note this as a deficiency.

HOUSING UNIT 131. Breakers/Fuses
(2003 IPMC CROSS-REFERENCE: 605.1 INSTALLATION)

DEFICIENCY: Breakers have carbon on the plastic body or the plastic body is melted or scarred.

NOTE: Do not attempt any disassembly of any electrical component or touch any circuit.

HOUSING UNIT 132. Water Leaks or Corrosion Near Electrical Systems
(2003 IPMC CROSS-REFERENCE: 605.1 INSTALLATION)

DEFICIENCY: There are liquid stains, rust marks, or other signs of corrosion on electrical enclosures or hardware.

NOTE: Do not consider surface rust a deficiency if it does not affect the condition of the electrical enclosure.

HOUSING UNIT 133. Wiring
(2003 IPMC CROSS-REFERENCE: 605.1 INSTALLATION)

DEFICIENCY: Electrical insulation is deteriorated.

HOUSING UNIT 134. Ground Fault Circuit Interrupter (GFCI)
(2003 IPMC CROSS-REFERENCE: 605.1 INSTALLATION)

DEFICIENCY: GFCI does not function or is missing. The model National Electrical Code requires GFCIs for electrical outlets in damp or wet locations. Examples include in bathrooms, in kitchens, in garages, near laundry sinks, and outdoors.

NOTE: To determine whether the GFCI is functioning, press the self-test button in the GFCI unit.

HOUSING UNIT 135. Arc Fault Circuit Interrupters
(2003 IPMC CROSS-REFERENCE: 605.1 INSTALLATION)

DEFICIENCY: AFCI does not function or is missing. Effective in 2002, the model National Electrical Code requires AFCIs for outlets in bedrooms.

HOUSING UNIT 136. Missing or Broken Electrical Covers
(2003 IPMC CROSS-REFERENCE: 605.1 INSTALLATION)

DEFICIENCY: In a panel board, main panel board, or other electrical box that contains circuit breakers/fuses, there is an open circuit breaker position that is not appropriately blanked-off-OR-The cover is missing from any electrical device box, panel box, switch gear box, control panel, etc., with exposed electrical connections.

HOUSING UNIT 137. Child Tamper-resistant Outlet Covers
(2003 IPMC CROSS-REFERENCE: NONE)

DEFICIENCY: Child tamper-resistant outlet covers are not installed in units where young children live.

HOUSING UNIT 138. Extension Cord Use
(2003 IPMC CROSS-REFERENCE: NONE)

DEFICIENCY: Extension cords are not used properly (are draped over doorways or under carpets) or are overloaded with multiple appliances.

HOUSING UNIT 139. Extension Cord Condition
(2003 IPMC CROSS-REFERENCE: NONE)

DEFICIENCY: Extension cords are cracked or frayed.

WATER HEATER

This inspectable item can have the following deficiencies: misaligned chimney/ventilation systems, inoperable unit/components, leaking valves/tanks/pipes, pressure relief valve missing, or rust/corrosion.

HOUSING UNIT 140. Water Heater Exhaust
(2003 IPMC CROSS-REFERENCES: 505.4 WATER HEATING FACILITIES; 603.2 REMOVAL OF COMBUSTION PRODUCTS)

DEFICIENCY: The exhaust system on a gas-fired or oil-fired hot water heater or heating unit is misaligned.

HOUSING UNIT 141. Water Temperature
(2003 IPMC CROSS-REFERENCE: 505.4 WATER HEATING FACILITIES)

DEFICIENCY: Hot water supply is not available because the system or system components have malfunctioned-OR-The temperature is set above 120°F-OR-There is no hot water.

HOUSING UNIT 142. Leaks
(2003 IPMC CROSS-REFERENCE: 505.4 WATER HEATING FACILITIES)

DEFICIENCY: Water is leaking from any hot water system component, including valve flanges, stems, bodies, or a domestic hot water tank or its piping.

HOUSING UNIT 143. Water Heater Temperature/Pressure Relief Valve
(2003 IPMC CROSS-REFERENCE: NONE)

DEFICIENCY: The temperature/pressure relief valve is missing.

NOTE: Do not operate the relief valve.

HOUSING UNIT 144. Water Heater Secured
(2003 IPMC CROSS-REFERENCE: NONE)

DEFICIENCY: The water heater is not strapped down to prevent tipping.

HVAC

Systems to provide heating, cooling and ventilation to the unit. This does not include building heating or cooling system deficiencies such as boilers, chillers, circulating pumps, distribution lines, fuel supply, etc., but does include ducts, radiators, baseboard heaters, etc.

This inspectable item can have the following deficiencies: convection/radiant heat system covers missing/damaged, general rust/corrosion, inoperable, misaligned chimney/ventilation systems, or noisy/vibrating/leaking.

HOUSING UNIT 145. General Rust/Corrosion (HVAC) Rust
(2003 IPMC CROSS-REFERENCE: 603.1 MECHANICAL APPLIANCES)

DEFICIENCY: A component of the HVAC system has deterioration from oxidation or corrosion of system parts.

HOUSING UNIT 146. HVAC Operation
(2003 IPMC CROSS-REFERENCE: 603.1 MECHANICAL APPLIANCES)

DEFICIENCY: The heating, cooling, or ventilation system does not function.

NOTE: If the HVAC system does not operate because of seasonal conditions, do not record it as a deficiency.

HOUSING UNIT 147. Supply Air for HVAC (From Basement Only)
(2003 IPMC CROSS-REFERENCE: NONE)

DEFICIENCY: All supply air for the HVAC system is drawn from the basement, with no functioning return air systems from living areas. Determine whether there is a source of fresh air delivered to the HVAC system (this does not include building leakage and/or open windows or doors).

HOUSING UNIT 148. HVAC Filters
(2003 IPMC CROSS-REFERENCE: NONE)

DEFICIENCY: HVAC filters are not clean (in equipment that requires filters).

HOUSING UNIT 149. HVAC Exhaust Ventilation System
(2003 IPMC CROSS-REFERENCE: 603.2 REMOVAL OF COMBUSTION PRODUCTS)

DEFICIENCY: The exhaust system on a fuel-fired unit is misaligned, damaged, blocked, or disconnected -OR-There is reversed air flow in the chimney/flue -OR-Rust or corrosion prevents the flue or exhaust systems from operating properly. **IF REVERSE AIR FLOW IS OBSERVED, REPORT TO BUILDING MANAGEMENT/OWNER IMMEDIATELY AND RECORD SPECIFICS IN THE COMMENTS SECTION.**

HOUSING UNIT 150. HVAC Noise
(2003 IPMC CROSS-REFERENCE: NONE)

DEFICIENCY: The HVAC distribution components, including fans, are the source of abnormal noise, unusual vibrations, or leaks.

HOUSING UNIT 151. Space Heaters
(2003 IPMC CROSS-REFERENCE: NONE)

DEFICIENCY: Space heaters used in unit are at not least 3 feet from anything that can burn.

HOUSING UNIT 152. Fireplace Screen
(2003 IPMC CROSS-REFERENCE: NONE)

DEFICIENCY: Fireplace does not have a sturdy screen to catch sparks

HOUSING UNIT 153. Fireplace Dampers
(2003 IPMC CROSS-REFERENCE: NONE)

DEFICIENCY: Fireplace dampers are not operational.

HOUSING UNIT 154. Wood Stove Barrier
(2003 IPMC CROSS-REFERENCE: NONE)

DEFICIENCY: There is no barrier in place to keep children away from wood stove surfaces.

KITCHEN
A place where food is cooked or prepared. The facilities and equipment used in preparing and serving food.

This inspectable item can have the following deficiencies: missing or damaged cabinets, countertops;

inoperable dishwasher or garbage disposal; clogged drains; leaking faucets or pipes; excessive grease or inoperable range hoods or exhaust fans; missing, damaged, or inoperable refrigerator, range, or stove; or missing or damaged sink.

HOUSING UNIT 155. Cabinets
(2003 IPMC CROSS-REFERENCE: NONE)

DEFICIENCY: Kitchen cabinets and/or their doors are missing. This includes cases, boxes, or pieces of furniture with drawers, shelves, or doors mounted on walls or floors and primarily used for storage.

HOUSING UNIT 156. Cabinet Damage

(2003 IPMC CROSS-REFERENCE: 305.3 INTERIOR SURFACES)

DEFICIENCY: Cabinets are damaged or not cleanable or have laminate separating on more than 20% of the surface

HOUSING UNIT 157. Countertops
(2003 IPMC CROSS-REFERENCE: NONE)

DEFICIENCY: A flat work surface in a kitchen, often integral to lower cabinet space, has laminate that is separating, or the surface is not smooth and cleanable.

HOUSING UNIT 158. Dishwasher
(2003 IPMC CROSS-REFERENCE: NONE)

DEFICIENCY: A dishwasher, if provided, does not function as it should.

HOUSING UNIT 159. Garbage Disposal
(2003 IPMC CROSS-REFERENCE: NONE)

DEFICIENCY: A garbage disposal, if provided, does not function as it should.

HOUSING UNIT 160. Kitchen Drain
(2003 IPMC CROSS-REFERENCE: 504.1 GENERAL)

DEFICIENCY: The water does not drain adequately.

HOUSING UNIT 161. Kitchen Plumbing
(2003 IPMC CROSS-REFERENCE: 504.1 GENERAL)

DEFICIENCY: A basin faucet or drain connection leaks -OR-There is visible mold.

HOUSING UNIT 162. Kitchen GFCI
(2003 IPMC CROSS-REFERENCE: NONE)

DEFICIENCY: No GFCI near the kitchen sink -OR-GFCI is near the sink but does not work properly. The model National Electrical Code requires GFCIs for electrical outlets in damp or wet locations—for example, in kitchens.

HOUSING UNIT 163. Water Temperature
(2003 IPMC CROSS-REFERENCE: NONE)

DEFICIENCY: Hot and cold water are not both present at kitchen plumbing fixtures.

HOUSING UNIT 164. Water Pressure
(2003 IPMC CROSS-REFERENCE: NONE)

DEFICIENCY: There is not adequate water pressure at all kitchen plumbing fixtures.

HOUSING UNIT 165. Range Hood
(2003 IPMC CROSS-REFERENCE: NONE)

DEFICIENCY: The apparatus that draws out cooking exhaust does not function as it should.

HOUSING UNIT 166. Range or Stove
(2003 IPMC CROSS-REFERENCE: 404.7 FOOD PREPARATION)

DEFICIENCY: The unit is missing or damaged.

HOUSING UNIT 167. Refrigerator
(2003 IPMC CROSS-REFERENCE: 404.7 FOOD PREPARATION)

DEFICIENCY: The refrigerator is missing or does not cool adequately for the safe storage of food.

HOUSING UNIT 168. Kitchen Sink
(2003 IPMC CROSS-REFERENCE: 504.1 GENERAL)

DEFICIENCY: A sink, faucet, or accessories are missing, damaged, or not functioning.

NOTE: If a stopper is missing, do not record it as a deficiency.

HOUSING UNIT 169. Permanent Carpet on Kitchen Floor

DEFICIENCY: Kitchen floor has permanent carpet or a noncleanable surface.

HOUSING UNIT 170. Cleaning Products

DEFICIENCY: Cleaning products are not stored out of the reach of children.

LAUNDRY AREA
Where soiled clothes and linens are washed and/or dried. This inspectable item can have the following deficiency: dryer vent missing, damaged, or inoperable.

HOUSING UNIT 171. Clothes Dryer
(2003 IPMC CROSS-REFERENCE: 403.5 CLOTHES DRYER EXHAUST)

DEFICIENCY: Clothes dryer is unable to vent accumulated heat/lint/moisture to the outside.

HOUSING UNIT 172. Exhaust Duct for Dryer
(2003 IPMC CROSS-REFERENCE: NONE)

DEFICIENCY: Flexible plastic or other combustible material is used for dryer exhaust ductwork.

HOUSING UNIT 173. Dryer Venting
(2003 IPMC CROSS-REFERENCE: NONE)

DEFICIENCY: Clothes dryer vents to basement, attic, or crawl space instead of outside.

LIGHTING

HOUSING UNIT 174. Interior Housing Unit Lighting
(2003 IPMC CROSS-REFERENCES: 402.2 COMMON HALLS AND STAIRWAYS; 402.3 OTHER SPACES; 605.3 LIGHTING FIXTURES)

Systems to provide illumination to a room or area. Includes fixtures, lamps, and supporting accessories. This inspectable item can have the following deficiency: missing/inoperable fixture.

DEFICIENCY: A lighting fixture is missing or does not function as it should. The malfunction may be in the total system or components, excluding light bulbs.

HOUSING UNIT 175. Outlets/Switches
(2003 IPMC CROSS-REFERENCE: 605.2 RECEPTACLES)

The receptacle connected to a power supply or method to control the flow of electricity. Includes two- and three-prong outlets, ground-fault circuit interrupters, pull cords, two- and three-pole switches, and dimmer switches. This inspectable item can have the following deficiencies: missing or missing/broken cover plates.

DEFICIENCY: An outlet, switch, or both are missing.

NOTE: This does not apply to empty junction boxes that were not intended to contain an outlet or switch.

PATIO/PORCH/BALCONY

HOUSING UNIT 176. Railings
(2003 IPMC CROSS-REFERENCE: 304.10 STAIRWAYS, DECKS, PORCHES AND BALCONIES)

Adjoining patio, porch, or balcony. This inspectable item can have the following deficiency: baluster/side railings damaged.

DEFICIENCY: A baluster or side railing on the porch/patio/balcony is loose, damaged, or does not function, limiting the safe use of this area.

HOUSING UNIT 177. Electrical Outlets
(2003 IPMC CROSS-REFERENCE: NONE)

DEFICIENCY: GFCIs are not present or are present but not functional. The model National Electrical Code requires GFCIs for electrical outlets in damp or wet locations—for example, outdoors.

HOUSING UNIT 178. Spindles and Railings

(2003 IPMC CROSS-REFERENCE: NONE)

DEFICIENCY: Spindles and railings are missing.

HOUSING UNIT 179. Spindles and Railings: Condition

(2003 IPMC CROSS-REFERENCE: NONE)

DEFICIENCY: Spindles and railings are damaged, loose, too low, or too far apart.

HOUSING UNIT 180. Spindles

(2003 IPMC CROSS-REFERENCE: NONE)

DEFICIENCY: Spindles are spaced more than 4 inches apart.

HOUSING UNIT 181. Railing Height

(2003 IPMC CROSS-REFERENCE: NONE)

DEFICIENCY: Railing is not between the recommended height of 30 and 42 inches.

HOUSING UNIT 182. Patio Surface

(2003 IPMC CROSS-REFERENCE: NONE)

DEFICIENCY: Patio surface has cracks with more than ¾ inch displacement.

SMOKE AND CARBON MONOXIDE DETECTORS

Sensor to detect the presence of smoke and/or carbon monoxide (CO) and activate an alarm. May be battery operated or hard-wired to electrical system. This inspectable item can have the following deficiency: missing/inoperable.

HOUSING UNIT 183. Smoke Detectors

(2003 IPMC CROSS-REFERENCE: 704.2 SMOKE ALARMS)

DEFICIENCY: No smoke detectors are present.

HOUSING UNIT 184. Smoke Detector Location

(2003 IPMC CROSS-REFERENCE: NONE)

DEFICIENCY: Smoke detectors are not located on every level of the home, in each bedroom, and in each common living area.

HOUSING UNIT 185. Smoke Detector Power

(2003 IPMC CROSS-REFERENCE: NONE)

DEFICIENCY: Smoke detectors are not powered by electricity with a battery backup.

HOUSING UNIT 186. Carbon Monoxide Detector

(2003 IPMC CROSS-REFERENCE: NONE)

DEFICIENCY: Carbon monoxide detectors are not present in a home with fuel-burning appliances and/or an attached garage.

HOUSING UNIT 187. CO Detector Location

(2003 IPMC CROSS-REFERENCE: NONE)

DEFICIENCY: There is not a CO detector near the bedroom area.

HOUSING UNIT 188. Fire Extinguisher

(2003 IPMC CROSS-REFERENCE: NONE)

DEFICIENCY: There is no charged fire extinguisher in the home.

STAIRS

Series of four or more steps or flights of steps joined by landings connecting levels of a unit. Includes supports, frame, treads, handrails. This inspectable item can have the following deficiencies: broken/missing hand railing or broken/damaged/missing steps.

HOUSING UNIT 189. Stair Railings

(2003 IPMC CROSS-REFERENCES: 305.4 STAIRS AND WALKING SURFACES; 305.5 HANDRAILS AND GUARDS; 306.1 GENERAL)

DEFICIENCY: The hand-rail is damaged or missing.

HOUSING UNIT 190. STEPS: Condition
(2003 IPMC CROSS-REFERENCE: 305.4 STAIRS AND WALKING SURFACES)

DEFICIENCY: The horizontal tread or stair surface is damaged or missing.

HOUSING UNIT 191. Steps: Covering
(2003 IPMC CROSS-REFERENCE: NONE)

DEFICIENCY: Stair covering (e.g., nonslip tread covers) is not firmly attached or is not in good condition.

WINDOWS
This inspectable item can have the following deficiencies: cracked/broken/missing panes, damaged window sill, inoperable/not lockable, missing/deteriorated caulking/seals, or peeling/needs paint.

HOUSING UNIT 192. Windows
(2003 IPMC CROSS-REFERENCE: 305.3 INTERIOR SURFACES)

DEFICIENCY: A glass pane is cracked, broken, or missing from the window sash.

HOUSING UNIT 193. Window Sills
(2003 IPMC CROSS-REFERENCE: 305.3 INTERIOR SURFACES)

DEFICIENCY: The sill (the interior horizontal part of the window that bears the upright portion of the frame) is damaged.

NOTE: When looking for damage to window sills, do not include scratches and cosmetic deficiencies.

HOUSING UNIT 194. Window Locks
(2003 IPMC CROSS-REFERENCE: 703.2 OPENING PROTECTIVES)

DEFICIENCY: A window cannot be opened or closed because of damage to the frame, faulty hardware, or another cause.

NOTE: If a window is not designed to lock, do not record this as a deficiency. Windows that are accessible from the outside—a ground-level window, for example—must be lockable.

HOUSING UNIT 195. Window Caulking/Seals
(2003 IPMC CROSS-REFERENCE: 305.3 INTERIOR SURFACES)

DEFICIENCY: The caulking or seals that resists weather is missing or deteriorated.

NOTE: This includes Thermopane and insulated windows that have failed. Caulk and seals are considered deteriorated when two or more seals for any window have lost their elasticity. (If the seals crumble and flake when touched, they have lost their elasticity.)

HOUSING UNIT 196. Window Paint
(2003 IPMC CROSS-REFERENCE: 305.3 INTERIOR SURFACES)

DEFICIENCY: Paint covering the window assembly or trim is cracking, flaking, or otherwise failing.

OTHER ITEMS (ITEMS 197–229)
Items to inspect in this category include
- Garbage and debris
- Injury hazards
- Childproofing measures
- Poisoning hazards
- Pest hazards
- Moisture hazards
- Swimming pool, spa, or whirlpool
- Other hazards

GARBAGE AND DEBRIS

OTHER 197. Indoors
(2003 IPMC CROSS-REFERENCE: 307.2.1 RUBBISH STORAGE FACILITIES)

DEFICIENCY: Too much garbage has gathered outside, more than the planned storage capacity -OR-Garbage has gathered in an area that is not sanctioned for staging or storing garbage or debris.

OTHER 198. Outdoors
(2003 IPMC CROSS-REFERENCE: 307.1 ACCUMULATION OF RUBBISH OR GARBAGE)

DEFICIENCY: Too much garbage has gathered, more than the planned storage capacity-OR-Garbage has gathered in an area that is not sanctioned for staging or storing garbage or debris.

INJURY HAZARDS

OTHER 199. Sharp Edges
(2003 IPMC CROSS-REFERENCE: NONE)

Physical hazards that pose risk for bodily injury. The following deficiencies can be noted: sharp edges or tripping.

DEFICIENCY: Physical defects (generally in commonly used or traveled areas) that could cause cutting or breaking human skin or other bodily harm.

OTHER 200. Trip Hazards
(2003 IPMC CROSS-REFERENCE: NONE)

DEFICIENCY: There are any physical defect that can pose a tripping risk (generally in walkways or other traveled areas).

OTHER 201. Garage Door Opener
(2003 IPMC CROSS-REFERENCE: NONE)

DEFICIENCY: The garage door does not reverse when it touches an object in its path.

CHILDPROOFING MEASURES

NOTE: These questions pertain to households where young children live or visit.

OTHER 202. Window Cords:
Strangulation Hazard
(2003 IPMC CROSS-REFERENCE: NONE)

DEFICIENCY: Looped window cords are present.

OTHER 203. Window Guards
(2003 IPMC CROSS-REFERENCE: NONE)

DEFICIENCY: There are no window guards.

OTHER 204. Cabinet Locks
(2003 IPMC CROSS-REFERENCE: NONE)

DEFICIENCY: Cabinet locks are not installed.

OTHER 205. Water Safety
(2003 IPMC CROSS-REFERENCE: NONE)

DEFICIENCY: Toilets are not covered (lids are not closed).

OTHER 206. Chemicals, Pesticides, Cleaning Supplies, or Medicines Stored Within Easy Reach of Children
(2003 IPMC CROSS-REFERENCE: NONE)

DEFICIENCY: Hazardous items—chemicals, pesticides, cleaning supplies, medicines—are not stored out of the reach of children.

OTHER 207. Hobbies
(2003 IPMC CROSS-REFERENCE: NONE)

DEFICIENCY: There is evidence of household hobbies that could pose a risk to young children.

POISONING HAZARDS

OTHER 208. Unvented Combustion Appliances Present
(2003 IPMC CROSS-REFERENCE: NONE)

DEFICIENCY: Fuel-fired combustion appliances, such as kerosene, LP gas, or other fuel-fired space heaters, generators, gas clothes driers, gas logs, stoves, ovens, charcoal grills etc., are used indoors without exhaust ventilation systems.

OTHER 209. Attached Garage
(2003 IPMC CROSS-REFERENCE: NONE)

DEFICIENCY: Attached garage is not sealed from the living area. The garage should be sealed against the passage of fire or toxic gases including carbon monoxide.

PEST HAZARDS

OTHER 210. INFESTATION: Roaches
(2003 IPMC CROSS-REFERENCE: 308.1 INFESTATION)
Presence of roaches.

DEFICIENCY: There is evidence of infestation of roaches throughout a unit or room, especially in food preparation and storage areas.

NOTE: If baits, traps, and sticky boards are present but show no presence of roaches, do not record this as a deficiency.

OTHER 211. Infestation: Rats or Mice
(2003 IPMC CROSS-REFERENCE: 302.5 RODENT HARBORAGE)

DEFICIENCY: There is evidence of rats or mice—sightings, rat or mouse holes, or droppings.

NOTE: If baits, traps, or sticky boards are present but show no presence of rats or mice, do not record this as a deficiency.

OTHER 212. Other Insects or Vermin
(2003 IPMC CROSS-REFERENCE: 308.1 INFESTATION)

DEFICIENCY: There is evidence of other insects or vermin (not roaches, mice, or rats); e.g., bats, birds, ants.

OTHER 213. Termite Tunnels
(2003 IPMC CROSS-REFERENCE: NONE)

DEFICIENCY: Active termite tunnels are present.

MOISTURE HAZARDS

OTHER 214. Sources of Excessive Humidity Present
(2003 IPMC CROSS-REFERENCE: NONE)

Sources of excessive humidity in homes include humidifiers, clothes dryers vented inside, and uncovered fish tanks).

OTHER 215. Moldy or Musty Odor Present
(2003 IPMC CROSS-REFERENCE: NONE)

DEFICIENCY: A moldy or musty odor is present.

OTHER 216. Dehumidifier Present
(2003 IPMC CROSS-REFERENCE: NONE)

DEFICIENCY: There is not a dehumidifier present but there should be one.

SWIMMING POOL, SPA, OR WHIRLPOOL

OTHER 217. Fencing and Gates
(2003 IPMC CROSS-REFERENCE: NONE)

DEFICIENCY: Fencing and gates for swimming pools, spas, or whirlpools are damaged or missing (or fence does not enclose on all four sides).

OTHER 218. Doors and Gates
(2003 IPMC CROSS-REFERENCE: NONE)

DEFICIENCY: Doors and gates for swimming pools, spas, or whirlpools do not close and latch automatically.

OTHER 219. Latches
(2003 IPMC CROSS-REFERENCE: NONE)

DEFICIENCY: Doors and gates for swimming pools, spas, or whirlpools do not have self-closing, self-latching devices at least 48 inches from the ground.

OTHER 220. Safety Equipment (Swimming Pool)
(2003 IPMC CROSS-REFERENCE: NONE)

DEFICIENCY: Life ring and shepherd's hook are not present in the swimming pool area.

OTHER 221. GFCI
(2003 IPMC CROSS-REFERENCE: NONE)

DEFICIENCY: No GFCI in swimming pool, spa, or whirlpool area-OR-GFCI present but not operational. The model National Electrical Code requires GFCIs for electrical outlets in damp or wet locations—for example, near swimming pools.

OTHER 222. Drain Cover
(2003 IPMC CROSS-REFERENCE: NONE)

DEFICIENCY: Drain cover missing or broken in swimming pool, spa, or whirlpool. **SHUT DOWN POOL, SPA, OR WHIRLPOOL IMMEDIATELY AND REPORT TO BUILDING MANAGEMENT/ OWNER. RECORD SPECIFICS IN THE COMMENTS SECTION.**

OTHER 223. Safety Cover (Spa)

(2003 IPMC CROSS-REFERENCE: NONE)

DEFICIENCY: Unlocked or missing safety cover on spa.

OTHER HAZARDS

OTHER 224. Visible Dust on Surfaces

(2003 IPMC CROSS-REFERENCE: NONE)

DEFICIENCY: There is heavy visible dust on surfaces.

OTHER 225. Air Cleaning Device Present

(2003 IPMC CROSS-REFERENCE: NONE)

DEFICIENCY: Not necessarily a deficiency; assessed because presence of an air-cleaning device could lead the inspector to other issues.

OTHER 226. Ozone Generator Present

(2003 IPMC CROSS-REFERENCE: NONE)

DEFICIENCY: There is an ozone generator present.

OTHER 227. Pets Present

(2003 IPMC CROSS-REFERENCE: NONE)

DEFICIENCY: Not necessarily a deficiency; assessed because presence of pets could lead the inspector to other issues.

OTHER 228. Tobacco Smoke or Odor Present

(2003 IPMC CROSS-REFERENCE: NONE)

DEFICIENCY: Tobacco smoke or odor is present.

OTHER 229. Other Hazards

(2003 IPMC CROSS-REFERENCE: NONE)

DEFICIENCY: There is evidence of any other hazards in or around the home (record in Comments and Notes).

COMMENTS AND NOTES

APPENDIX 2:
2003 INTERNATIONAL PROPERTY MAINTENANCE CODE (2003 IPMC) CROSS-REFERENCES

The 2003 International Property Maintenance Code addresses maintenance requirements for structures, including requirements for heating, plumbing, lighting, and ventilation in existing residences.

The 2003 IPMC is available for adoption and use by jurisdictions worldwide.

Copies of the 2003 IPMC can be ordered from the International Code Council (ICC): http://www.iccsafe.org/e/category.html or 1-800-786-4452.

2003 IPMC CODE PROVISIONS

300
301.3   Vacant structures and land

302
302.1   Sanitation
302.2   Grading and drainage
302.3   Sidewalks and driveways
302.4   Weeds
302.5   Rodent harborage
302.6   Exhaust vents
302.7   Accessory structures
302.8   Motor vehicles
302.9   Defacement of property

303
303.1   Swimming pools
303.2   Enclosures

304
304.1   General [exterior structure]
304.10 Stairways, decks, porches and balconies
304.11 Chimneys and towers
304.12 Handrails and guards
304.13 Window, skylight and door frames
304.13.1   Glazing
304.13.2   Openable windows
304.14 Insect screens
304.15 Doors
304.16 Basement hatchways
304.17 Guards for basement windows
304.18 Building security
304.18.1   Doors
304.18.2   Windows
304.18.3   Basement hatchways

304.2   Protective treatment
304.3   Premises identification
304.4   Structural members
304.5   Foundation walls
304.6   Exterior walls
304.7   Roofs and drainage
304.8   Decorative features
304.9   Overhang extensions

305
305.1   General [interior structure]
305.2   Structural members
305.3   Interior surfaces
305.4   Stairs and walking surfaces
305.5   Handrails and guards
305.6   Interior doors

306
306.1   General [stairs]

307
307.1   Accumulation of rubbish or garbage
307.2   Disposal of rubbish
307.2.1 Rubbish storage facilities
307.2.2 Refrigerators
307.3   Disposal of garbage
307.3.1 Garbage facilities
307.3.2 Containers

308
308.1   Infestation

APPENDIX 3:
ADDITIONAL RESOURCES
OPTIONAL ENVIRONMENTAL SAMPLING METHODS: LINKS TO INFORMATION ON THE INTERNET

Environmental sampling for contaminants can sometimes yield additional useful information on housing related health hazards. Each sampling method has its strengths and weaknesses, inherent sampling and analytical error and interferences. Multiple methods exist to sample each contaminant. Sampling must be performed carefully, properly, and in a manner that protects both the person doing the sampling and the occupants. Instruments for certain contaminants may be able to measure the contaminant in real time. For some substances, sampling in the home environment may require a license or certification or training or other requirements in certain jurisdictions.

Consult your local or state government to determine whether such requirements apply before undertaking any environmental sampling in the home environment. If laboratory analysis is required, consult with the analytic laboratory before collecting any sample. If you are uncertain about how to use a particular method or have not been trained, it is recommended that you consult with the local health or environmental department, a professional industrial hygienist or other environmental scientist.

This list of methods and products is not intended to be exhaustive. Additional or other sampling procedures may be recommended in any individual situation. Use of detector tubes and any instrumentation must always be performed according to the manufacturer's instructions. Listing in this document is not intended to be an endorsement of any product or method by the National Center for Healthy Housing or any government agency.

AGENCY/ORGANIZATION KEY	
ALA	American Lung Association
AWWA	American Water Works Association
CPSC	Consumer Product Safety Commission
NIH	National Institutes of Health
NPS	National Park Servcie
NSC	National Safety Council
NSFC	National Small Flows Clearinghouse
U.S. EPA	Environmental Protection Agency
UL	Underwriters Laboratory
USDA	U.S. Department of Agriculture
USFA	U.S. Fire Administration
USGS	U.S. Geological Survey

ASBESTOS BULK SAMPLING

http://www.epa.gov/region9/toxic/noa/eldorado/pdf/NIOSH9002.pdf

CARBON DIOXIDE (DETECTOR TUBE)

http://www.skcshopping.com/ProductDetails.asp?ProductCode=810-2LL

CARBON MONOXIDE (DETECTOR TUBE)

http://www.skcshopping.com/ProductDetails.asp?ProductCode=810-1LL

COCKROACHES

http://www.cehrc.org/docUploads/CEHRC_Cockroaches_Materials.pdf

FORMALDEHYDE (DETECTOR TUBE)

http://www.skcshopping.com/ProductDetails.asp?ProductCode=810-91LL

LEAD IN PAINT CHIPS

Appendix 13.2 in the HUD Guidelines, http://www.hud.gov/offices/lead/guidelines/hudguidelines/Appendix.pdf

LEAD IN PAINT BY X-RAY FLUORESCENCE
http://www.hud.gov/offices/lead/guidelines/
hudguidelines/Chap7_2.pdf

LEAD IN SETTLED HOUSE DUST
Appendix 13.1, http://www.hud.gov/offices/lead/
guidelines/hudguidelines/Appendix.pdf

LEAD IN SOIL
Appendix 13.3, http://www.hud.gov/offices/lead/
guidelines/hudguidelines/Appendix.pdf

OZONE (DETECTOR TUBE)
http://www.skcshopping.com/ProductDetails.
asp?ProductCode=810-18L

RADON
http://www.epa.gov/radon/methods.html

SELECTED WEB REFERENCES FOR HEALTHY HOMES ISSUES

The National Center for Healthy Housing offers training for individuals and organizations interested in healthy housing issues, including lead poisoning prevention, methods for lead hazard control, integrated pest management, and radon education: http://healthyhomestraining.org.

The CDC/HUD Healthy Housing Reference Manual is online at http://www.cdc.gov/nceh/publications/books/housing/housing.htm. Hard copies and CD-ROM versions can be ordered by calling 1-800-CDC-INFO or sending an e-mail to cdcinfo@cdc.gov.

ANTISCALDING DEVICES
HUD, http://www.hud.gov/offices/lead/hhi/
HHIInjury_3-29-2002.pdf

CPSC, http://www.cpsc.gov/cpscpub/pubs/
grand/12steps/12steps.html

ASBESTOS
U.S. EPA, http://www.epa.gov/iaq/asbestos.html

U.S. EPA, www.epa.gov/asbestos/ashome.html
Oklahoma State University, http://www.pp.okstate.
edu/ehs/links/asbestos.htm

BATS
CDC, http://www.cdc.gov/ncidod/dvrd/rabies/bats_&_
rabies/bats&.htm
Illinois Department of Public Health, http://www.
idph.state.il.us/public/hb/hbb&bdrp.htm

USGS, http://www.npwrc.usgs.gov/resource/1998/
housebat/public.htm

BEDBUGS
NPS, http://www.nps.gov/public_health/intra/info/
factsheets/fs_bed_bugs_gen.pdf

New Mexico State University, http://cahe.nmsu.edu/
pubs/_g/g-318.html

CARBON MONOXIDE
CDC, http://www.cdc.gov/co/

HUD, http://www.hud.gov/offices/lead/helpyourself/
Carbon.pdf

CPSC, http://www.cpsc.gov/cpscpub/pubs/466.html

U.S. EPA, http://www.epa.gov/iaq/co.html

CHILDPROOFING AND BABYPROOFING
HUD, http://healthyhomestraining.org/Documents/
HUD/HUD_Home_Safety_FS.pdf

U.S. EPA, http://www.epa.gov/pesticides/factsheets/
childsaf.htm

CSPC, http://cpsc.gov/

COCKROACHES
CDC, http://www.cdc.gov/nasd/docs/
d001201-d001300/d001251/d001251.pdf

HUD, http://ehw.org/Asthma/ASTH_HUDRoach_
Sum.htm

U.S. EPA, http://www.epa.gov/asthma/pests.html

U.S. EPA, http://es.epa.gov/ncer/childrenscenters/
controllingpest.html

ELECTRICAL SAFETY

CSPC, http://www.cpsc.gov/cpscpub/pubs/elec_sfy.html

ENVIRONMENTAL TOBACCO SMOKE

CDC, http://www.cdc.gov/tobacco/data_statistics/Factsheets/SecondhandSmoke.htm

U.S. EPA, http://www.epa.gov/smokefree/publications.html

FIRE PREVENTION

CDC, http://www.cdc.gov/ncipc/factsheets/fireprevention.htm

CSPC, http://www.cpsc.gov/cpscpub/pubs/fire_sfy.html

Public-Private Fire Safety Council, http://www.firesafety.gov

USFA, http://www.usfa.dhs.gov/citizens/

FIREPLACES AND RADIANT HEATERS

CDC, http://www.cdc.gov/nasd/docs/d001201-d001300/d001235/d001235.html

U.S. EPA, http://www.epa.gov/woodstoves/

USFA, http://www.usfa.dhs.gov/citizens/

USFA, http://www.usfa.dhs.gov/citizens/all_citizens/home_fire_prev/heating/index.shtm

FOOD SAFETY

CDC, http://www.cdc.gov/foodsafety/

HUD, http://www.hud.gov/offices/lead/helpyourself/Pest.pdf

U.S. EPA, http://www.epa.gov/ebtpages/pestpesticfoodsafety.html

USDA, http://www.foodsafety.gov

GARAGE DOOR SAFETY

CPSC, http://www.cpsc.gov/CPSCPUB/PUBS/523.html

UL, http://www.ul.com/consumers/garagedoors.html

HOME HEATING SAFETY

CDC, http://www.cdc.gov/nasd/docs/d001201-d001300/d001235/d001235.html

U.S. EPA, http://www.epa.gov/iaq/co.html

U.S. EPA, http://www.epa.gov/woodstoves/

USFA, http://www.usfa.dhs.gov/citizens/

USFA, http://www.usfa.dhs.gov/citizens/all_citizens/home_fire_prev/heating/index.shtm

CPSC, http://www.cpsc.gov/cpscpub/pubs/466.html

HUMIDIFIER SAFETY

U.S. EPA, http://www.epa.gov/iaq/pubs/humidif.html

CPSC, http://www.cpsc.gov/CPSCPUB/PUBS/5046.html

KITCHEN SAFETY

CDC, http://www.cdc.gov/nasd/docs/d000801-d000900/d000825/d000825.html

FDA, http://www.foodsafety.gov

NSC, http://www.nsc.org/news/nr112105b.htm

LEAD AND LEAD DUST

CDC, www.cdc.gov/nceh/lead/lead.htm

HUD, http://www.hud.gov/offices/lead/

U.S. EPA, www.epa.gov/opptintr/lead

U.S. EPA, http://www.epa.gov/ttn/atw/hlthef/lead.html

MICE

CDC, http://www.cdc.gov/rodents/

U.S. EPA, http://es.epa.gov/ncer/childrenscenters/controllingpest.html

MOLD

CDC, http://www.cdc.gov/mold/

HUD, http://www.hud.gov/offices/lead/prevention.cfm

U.S. EPA, http://www.epa.gov/iaq/molds/moldcleanup.html

U.S. EPA, http://www.epa.gov/iaq/molds/moldbasics.html

PESTICIDE SAFETY

HUD, http://www.hud.gov/offices/lead/helpyourself/Pest.pdf

U.S. EPA, http://www.epa.gov/pesticides/health/index.htm

NIH, http://www.nlm.nih.gov/medlineplus/pesticides.html

RADON

CDC, http://www.cdc.gov/nceh/radiation/brochure/profile_radon.htm

HUD, http://www.hud.gov/offices/lead/helpyourself/Air.pdf

U.S. EPA, http://www.epa.gov/iaq/pubs/sbs.html

ALA, http://www.lungusa.org/site/pp.asp?c=dvLUK9O0E&b=35420

RATS

CDC, http://www.cdc.gov/rodents/

U.S. EPA, http://es.epa.gov/ncer/childrenscenters/controllingpest.html

NPS, http://www.nature.nps.gov/biology/ipm/manual/rats.cfm

SEPTIC TANKS/ONSITE WASTEWATER TREATMENT SYSTEMS

CDC, http://www.cdc.gov/nceh/ehs/topics/wastewater.htm

HUD, http://www.hudclips.org/sub_nonhud/cgi/nph-brs.cgi?d=HSGA&s1=4145.1&l=100&SECT1=TXT_HITS&SECT5=HEHB&u=./hudclips.cgi&p=1&r=48&f=G

U.S. EPA, http://cfpub.epa.gov/owm/septic/index.cfm

U.S. EPA, http://www.epa.gov/safewater/mcl.html#mcls

NSFC, http://www.nesc.wvu.edu/nsfc/

SLIPS AND FALLS

CDC, http://www.cdc.gov/ncipc/

SPRING WATER FOR DRINKING

U.S. EPA, http://www.epa.gov/OGWDW/

AWWA, http://www.awwa.org/

SWIMMING POOL, SPA, AND WHIRLPOOL SAFETY

CDC, http://www.cdc.gov/healthyswimming

CPSC, http://www.cpsc.gov/cpscpub/pubs/chdrown.html

WATER FILTRATION SYSTEMS

U.S. EPA, http://www.epa.gov/safewater

U.S. EPA, http://www.epa.gov/safewater/contaminants/index.html

UL, http://www.ULDrinkWell.com

WELL WATER FOR DRINKING

U.S. EPA, http://www.epa.gov/safewater

UL, http://www.ULDrinkWell.com

www.ingramcontent.com/pod-product-compliance
Lightning Source LLC
Chambersburg PA
CBHW080309180526
45167CB00006B/2729